PARTNERSHIP
of EQUALS

PRACTICAL STRATEGIES FOR HEALTHCARE

CEOs AND THEIR BOARDS

PARTNERSHIP
of EQUALS

PRACTICAL STRATEGIES FOR HEALTHCARE

CEOs AND THEIR BOARDS

PETER McGINN

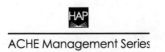

ACHE Management Series

Your board, staff, or clients may also benefit from this book's insight. For more information on quantity discounts, contact the Health Administration Press Marketing Manager at (312) 424-9470.

This publication is intended to provide accurate and authoritative information in regard to the subject matter covered. It is sold, or otherwise provided, with the understanding that the publisher is not engaged in rendering professional services. If professional advice or other expert assistance is required, the services of a competent professional should be sought.

The statements and opinions contained in this book are strictly those of the author(s) and do not represent the official positions of the American College of Healthcare Executives or of the Foundation of the American College of Healthcare Executives.

Copyright © 2009 by the Foundation of the American College of Healthcare Executives. Printed in the United States of America. All rights reserved. This book or parts thereof may not be reproduced in any form without written permission of the publisher.

Reprinted September 2018

Library of Congress Cataloging-in-Publication Data

Partnership of equals: practical strategies for healthcare CEOs and their boards/by
    Peter McGinn.
        p. ; cm.
Includes bibliographical references.
ISBN-13: 978-1-56793-311-6
ISBN-10: 1-56793-311-4
1. Health facilities—Administration. 2. Chief executive officers. 3. Hospital
    administrators. 4. Hospital trustees. I. Title.
[DNLM: 1. Administrative Personnel. 2. Health Care Reform—organization &
    administration. 3. Consultants. 4. Governing Board. WA 525 M4775c 2009]
RA971.M248 2009
362.11068′3—dc22
                                                            2008041475

Find an error or typo? We want to know! Please e-mail it to HAP1@ache.org, and put "Book Error" in the subject line.

Photocopying and Copyright Information
Please contact Copyright Clearance Center at www.copyright.com or 978-750-8400.

The paper used in this publication meets the minimum requirements of American National Standard for Information Sciences—Permanence of Paper for Printed Library Materials, ANSI Z39.48-1984.™

Acquisitions editor: Janet Davis; Project manager: Dojna Shearer;
Book designer: Scott Miller; Composition: Putman Productions, LLC.

Health Administration Press
A division of the Foundation of the
American College of Healthcare Executives
1 North Franklin Street, Suite 1700
Chicago, IL 60606-3529
(312) 424-2800

CONTENTS

ACKNOWLEDGMENTS

Writing is considered a lonely occupation. Franz Kafka said, "Writing is utter solitude, the descent into the cold abyss of oneself." That, like Kafka himself, is a bit extreme, but it does reflect the general attitude toward writing. However, although I spent many hours by myself writing and rewriting, the development of this book was also a very social experience. I shared the chapters as I wrote them with colleagues from coast to coast, and even around the world. I received their support, encouragement, comments, questions, and suggestions. I may have been working in quiet solitude a lot of the time, but I never felt alone.

Don Carlin, Lynne Cunningham, Steve Goldstein, and Paul Hofmann, PhD, read almost the entire book as I was writing it and helped me sharpen my thinking and clarify my writing. Others who provided helpful advice or reviewed various chapters include: Akram Boutros, MD; Eric Brown; Keith Fenstemacher; Mike Fuller; Frank Gilroy, MD; Lee Golden; Patrick Hayes; Kerry Luse, PhD; Kathryn McGinn; Mark O'Neil; Keith Pryor; Vasanti Rao, MD; Art Ricchiuti; Virender Sangwan, MD; John Stack; Mark Stensager; Mike Ueltzen; Jerry Vasile, PhD; and Alan Zuckerman. It goes without saying that I also benefited throughout from past experiences with my former colleagues and boards at

United Health Services and from my current consulting engagements with boards and senior teams in client health systems and other for-profit and not-for-profit organizations. I offer special thanks to my three board chairs, Frank Gilroy, MD; James Lee, PhD; and Judith Peckham. Please do not hold any of the above liable, however, for errors or ambiguities that may remain. I take sole responsibility for those.

Once again in writing a book for Health Administration Press, I had the pleasure of working with a talented and supportive team of editors and staff including Janet Davis, acquisitions editor, and Dojna Shearer, project manager.

Finally, I want to take the opportunity to acknowledge the constant support of my wife, Marilyn McGinn, and to dedicate this book to her. She has been my partner for 38 years. Anyone who has been a CEO, a board member, a consultant, or an author knows how important the unconditional love and support of a spouse is. Since I have been all four, sometimes simultaneously, I treasure her constant help and encouragement. That was one more way in which I was never alone.

INTRODUCTION

Many CEOs consider their boards a necessary evil, a fact of life to
be accommodated but not embraced. Others look to their boards
as community advocates, fundraisers, and sounding boards, but
not as their superiors. Some reflect on management excesses else-
where and conclude that boards constitute a protection for the
assets of society and as such are necessary in general, even if not
actually required in their own specific settings. Finally, some
CEOs develop a sense of partnership with their boards. They
view board members as sharing their commitment to the organization's mission and seek to employ the talents, connections, and
perspectives of the board just as they employ the skills, motivation, and energies of staff to make decisions and get things done.
An ineffective board undermines the efforts of staff, but a good
board makes a CEO and an organization better. As a consultant
and former healthcare CEO, I recognize these varying attitudes in
my colleagues because, over the years, I have held each attitude at
one time or another.

CEOs know that the board cycle is one of the drumbeats that
establishes the rhythm of work in not-for-profit organizations.
Preparing for board meetings consumes a substantial percentage
of a CEO's time. Other work takes second place as scheduled

board meetings move closer. When board members make requests (or demands), CEOs respond. Some CEOs seek to ensure job security by making the care and feeding of board members their top priority. The responsibility for board relations constitutes one of the biggest role shifts as an executive moves into the CEO position. It is a job the CEO cannot delegate.

A CEO must find a way to come to terms with such a dominant feature on the organizational landscape. If the board is an obstacle, how can its impact be minimized? If it is an asset, how can its impact be multiplied? And if it can be either, how can its impact be optimized?

The *politically correct* position is that boards are assets. In this view, things work in reality just as they are supposed to in theory. That is, boards deliberate, set direction, establish policy, hire their chief executives, and delegate authority to them for management. Clashes between boards and executives are symptoms of role definition flaws or of personality or skill deficits of individuals. If everyone just knows and accepts his or her role, 90 percent of the problems will fade away. If each party stays on the correct side of the management–governance divide, and if board chairs and CEOs each devote sufficient time to board development, then goodwill and harmony will reign.

I, on the other hand, take a more pragmatic stance, based on experience and understanding of human nature. Boards can be obstacles or assets. The legal structure and the traditional allocation of board and CEO responsibilities are in part products of history, court decisions, corporate models, and other random factors. Layered on top of this are the individual personalities, histories, philosophies, strengths, and flaws of board members and CEOs. Some are well-meaning, personally secure, and mature, but not all. Some are up to the challenges and tasks of leadership, but not all. Some have had intelligent instruction and good role models, but not all. Some are passionate about mission rather than about personal opportunities, but not all. As Yogi Berra reportedly said: "In theory, theory and practice are the same. In practice, they are different."

I joined my first board, the Mental Health Association of Metropolitan Baltimore, when I was in my early 20s. I considered it an honor, but I had no concept of the fiduciary responsibilities I had assumed. A few years later, shortly after President Nixon resigned because of the Watergate scandal, I accepted a position as a staff member in the U.S. Senate. The tensions between the legislative and executive branches, which had always been present in DC, grew to enormous proportions. After leaving Washington, I became a candidate for the school board in a small Michigan town. I ran on a reform platform, opposing the district superintendent, and was elected. That put me into direct opposition to the sitting administration. Both in Washington and in Michigan, I experienced the basic relationship between executive and legislature/board as one of suspicion and conflict—not a very balanced preparation for the responsibilities I would later assume, where trust and collaboration were essential.

Later I became a vice president in a newly formed health system, providing staff support to the board and CEO. We worked through crisis situations and recruited new CEOs in a couple of the system's organizations. These experiences further shaped my understanding of the board's role. I came to see a more positive and constructive relationship between boards and administrators. They worked together on behalf of the mission and business of the health system. I also observed, however, two imbalances: The board had final authority, but administration had more content knowledge and generally established the agenda. Thus, while the board possessed legal power, management exercised practical power.

My education continued when I became CEO of that health system. I served on the system board and as an officer of each of the subsidiary boards. I also served as chair of the state hospital association board and all of its subsidiaries. I learned from my colleagues and from board experts, read about boards, and attended meetings and conferences that described and prescribed board and CEO relations. I also learned from experience that what is in the books does not adequately capture the practical realities on the ground. As CEO, I sought to build a working partnership with boards that was functional for the organization and met the legal requirements.

How can the impact of the board be optimized, taking into account that boards, board members, *and* CEOs can perform either effectively or ineffectively? I have faced this issue both as a CEO and as a board member, and I will address it in this book. I intend to suggest a new metaphor for the board–CEO relationship that I believe will help CEOs improve the effectiveness of boards: I recommend that CEOs emulate the behavior of consultants when dealing with their boards. The legal relationship of boards and CEOs would not change with this new attitude, just the practical realities of their respective roles.

In a consultant–client relationship, the client hires the consultant, and the consultant works at the pleasure of the client. The consultant normally possesses some knowledge or skills that the client does not have. The consultant advises the client, makes suggestions, and offers assistance, but the client is responsible for making decisions. The client may hire the consultant to do some work, identify desired outcomes, and set parameters, but would not normally tell the consultant how to do the work. There are differences in the roles of client and consultant, but there is a significant level of parity as well. It is an adult–adult relationship. Clients and consultants each need to explicitly outline their expectations rather than simply assuming they expect the same thing. When the two parties get out of sync, they need to work through the disharmony as partners.

CEOs are not actually consultants, nor are boards really clients. Consultants seldom have the deep, lasting emotional commitment to their clients that CEOs have to their organizations. Consultants do not have delegated authority for *running* the organization except in limited circumstances, such as a bankruptcy restructuring.

However, the metaphor enables one to look at board–CEO relationships as partnerships of equals who use their skills and insights on behalf of their organizations. In a practical day-to-day sense, the metaphor establishes boards as having the ultimate power and authority without implying a parent–child relationship. It removes the question of whether boards are obstacles or assets; consultants do not ask whether their clients are obstacles or assets.

In the material that follows, I will use the consultant metaphor to offer practical advice for CEOs and board members who are seeking to improve their relationships and organizational performance. If you find a conflict between what I suggest and what you understand the legal requirements to be, seek appropriate advice and follow your understanding of the legal requirements. I will be surprised if such a circumstance arises, as I do not believe my recommendations will be at odds with the legal perspective. I do intend, however, to offer different perspectives that should help you look at your challenges and opportunities with fresh eyes.

I have structured this book around three main questions:

1. Who should be on the board?
2. What does the board do?
3. How should the board do it?

Each of these topics forms one of the principle sections of the book, although the separation is a bit arbitrary as the topics naturally intertwine. Each section includes four or five short chapters focusing on the practical problems and issues CEOs and boards deal with most often or find the most challenging. Each chapter concludes with a set of application guidelines for the CEO and a companion set for board members.

Section I ("Who?") covers board membership, physician members of boards, the chair and the executive committee, and CEO selection and succession. Section II ("What?") includes chapters on setting direction, establishing and maintaining standards, board appraisal and development, CEO appraisal and development, and managing problems and crises. Section III ("How?") focuses on relationships, board meetings, maximizing participation, and making decisions. In addition to the three primary sections, one more chapter covers system and subsidiary boards and the implications for CEO–board relations in that context. I conclude with a summary chapter that reprises the core themes of the book and urges CEOs and boards to stay focused on mission, strategy, and the road ahead.

I intend this book for both management and board members in healthcare, but the primary audience is CEOs. They experience and understand best the problems and deficiencies inherent in the usual management–board relations. However, I want to encourage CEOs to put this book into the hands of their board members. I want both parties to be fully aware of the opportunities that open to them when the process works better. I expect most board members who read this book will receive it from CEOs who wish to elevate the board–CEO relationship and increase the effectiveness and impact of their boards.

Although I've written this book for a healthcare audience, I believe that CEOs and boards in other not-for-profit organizations will also find great applicability. They face many of the same challenges as their counterparts in healthcare, even if the details differ. Finally, I expect that senior managers other than CEOs will find the descriptions in this book useful as an explanation of a key dynamic in the organization's life.

Boards and CEOs can work together to accomplish great things, but to do that, they need to get out of common governance ruts and allow their strengths to shine.

SECTION I

WHO?

CHAPTER 1

BOARD SELECTION

Some CEOs try to pack their boards with their friends or allies. Others defer completely to their boards on the question of selection. Board selection is properly the province of the board, but the CEO should not take a hands-off approach. A CEO who does that is missing a great opportunity to aid the board in its work. On the other hand, a CEO who stacks the board is undoubtedly subverting the board's authority and independence and likely limiting its overall quality and diversity.

What would a CEO do if he or she were consulting the board? A consultant would look at the challenges the board faces and is likely to confront in the future and would advise the board regarding criteria and candidates that would serve its needs and the community best. This means the CEO must be deeply engaged in the process, taking the long view and carefully analyzing alternatives.

I once served on the board of a troubled, not-for-profit hospital. Because of errors, bad luck, and a difficult environment, the hospital had found itself on shaky financial ground. It had lost the community's confidence. Serving on the board required a deep commitment to the hospital's community mission.

When it came time to replace retiring board members with new ones, the obvious candidates in the community demurred when offered the opportunity to serve, because of the magnitude of the hospital's problems. The governance committee then dug a little deeper and developed a second slate of candidates. Each of them, in turn, passed on the opportunity, for the same reasons. The committee persisted. It looked beyond the usual candidates and identified several potential nominees who would not typically have been sought out for board positions. I was delighted. These candidates were more diverse than the initial two sets, they had deeper allegiance to the community, and they felt privileged to serve. The board strengthened itself in ways that would have been unlikely if it had been able to recruit its first choices.

For me, this experience provided three lessons. First, greater diversity and talent were available than had initially appeared. Second, we should not have waited until crisis struck to undertake efforts to strengthen the board. Third, the CEO and the board could have, and should have, been cultivating some of these unrecognized potential board members far in advance of the impending retirement of the outgoing board members.

GETTING THE RIGHT PEOPLE ON BOARD

In *Good to Great*, Jim Collins (2001, 41–42) describes the concept of "first who, then what." Here is how he puts it:

> The executives who ignited the transformations from good to great did not first figure out where to drive the bus and then get people to take it there. No, they first got the right people on the bus (and the wrong people off the bus) and then figured out where to drive it. . . . [I]f you have the right people on the bus, the problem of how to motivate and manage people largely goes away. The right people don't need to be tightly managed or fired up; they will be self-motivated by

the inner drive to produce the best results and to be part of creating something great. . . . Great vision without great people is irrelevant.

A board and CEO who follow Collins's advice will understand that they must get the right board members on the bus in addition to hiring the right employees. If the wrong people are on your board, they may actually impede your progress and draw you off course. As the body that approves budgets, plans, and policies, an ineffective board will undermine the performance of even the most talented and committed staff. An effective board, however, can open new doors, sponsor innovation, and accelerate growth and development. Therefore, the selection of board members will influence every other activity down the road.

THE CROSSWORD PUZZLE

Selecting the right board members is like completing a crossword puzzle. In a crossword, each word fills a special need (solves a clue) while simultaneously interlinking with several other words. Each word solved becomes, in turn, a partial clue for other words. No word stands by itself; each one has meaning and makes a special contribution to the solution of the whole puzzle. In some cases, an individual word becomes a key that unlocks the theme of the puzzle by how it leads to recognizing patterns in the other clues and solutions. Boards work the same way. No individual board member can do the work of the whole board. The interrelationships among the members create a dynamic energy that furthers the board's work. In some cases, individual members become catalysts who energize other board members.

A CEO who is consulting with the board on the identification and selection of members should keep this metaphor in mind. Just as no one would expect a crossword puzzle to be solved by using the same word over and over, no one should expect a great board to consist of clones. Because homogeneity of members may occur if board members recruit new members who are friends and colleagues, a CEO can enrich the process by uncovering candidates who might otherwise be overlooked.

Most boards find it useful to create a skills and attributes grid to summarize skills possessed by board members and to identify skills or attributes it will seek when it recruits new members. A common mistake, however, is to specify skills needed for managing the organization. Except for new or small not-for-profits, such an approach can mislead the board and actually set the stage for board and management roles to become blurred. It is desirable to recruit people with good business and financial skills because of the judgment and perspective they can bring to board deliberations, not so they can act as unpaid technical advisers or doers. Think about skills broadly and at a high level of analysis rather than as functional responsibilities.

PASSION AND SKILLS

Here is an important qualifier. Whatever other types of criteria may be established for board positions, two are essential: skill and passion for the mission of the organization. Consider Table 1.1.

Occasionally a board or a CEO may be tempted to overlook one factor or the other, figuring skills can be developed or passion can be nurtured. Sometimes the gamble pays off, but there should be no doubt that it is an expensive gamble. Economists have coined the term *opportunity cost* to describe this. Whenever a less desirable alternative is chosen, the cost of that alternative includes the missed benefits of the choice not made. Because board seats are limited in number, any weak board members cost not only in terms of the errors or impediments they generate, but also in terms of losing the contributions of potentially more productive board members. As consultant to the board, the CEO should help the board avoid this common error.

Table 1.1 Passion and Skills Are Essential Qualities of a Board Member

	Low Passion for Mission	High Passion for Mission
High Skills	Talented but uncommitted. Contributes to the work of the board, but potentially disruptive.	Talented and dependable. Will sacrifice individual goals for the goals of the organization. Valuable in a crisis.
Low Skills	A board member in name but not in deed. May be looking for what can be gotten from the board, not what can be contributed. Impairs the work of the board and occupies a slot that could be better filled by someone else.	Loyal and dependable but does not add to the board process and may take the board off course on occasion. Loses credibility over time, so others may overlook valid contributions.

CULTIVATING BOARD MEMBERS

The CEO should act as a talent scout for the board. Part of the CEO's role in the community involves developing a network of relationships from which board members are likely to be recruited. When board vacancies develop, a prepared CEO will have become familiar with a broad range of possible candidates. Under the best circumstances, the CEO will have already evaluated potential board members through informal discussions and observations. In addition, the CEO will have shared enough about the organization and its mission to stimulate candidates' interest and get a reading on their reactions.

Candidates who raise relevant questions or who inquire about the organization's actions and challenges are sending positive signals. Those who demonstrate an interest in the larger political and economic environment as it affects healthcare are demonstrating an intelligent awareness of context. Likewise, those who make comparisons to their own challenges and experiences show that they are thinking beyond the surface and making connections. Individuals who have been successful in their own businesses or careers often bring perspectives and judgment that are reflected in the ways they understand issues and grasp implications.

The CEO, in turn, should be sharing more about the vision of the organization and describing problems that challenge the board, management, and staff. As time goes on, the CEO lets the prospective candidate in on things that happen behind the scenes, providing a view that is not normally seen by outsiders—excluding, of course, information that is confidential or proprietary. Each of these steps helps the CEO gauge the skills and passion of the potential board member. This cultivation process helps nurture interest in participating on the board.

When the nominating or governance committee meets to consider possible candidates, the CEO will be able to serve as a knowledgeable partner. The CEO can suggest possible board members and can comment helpfully on many of those raised as prospects by other board members. By doing so, the CEO is likely to stimulate more ideas, perspectives, and options by the members of the committee. The CEO is not controlling the process, but rather is seeding it in a way that builds the confidence of the board and increases the likelihood of good outcomes.

APPLICATION GUIDELINES FOR THE CEO

1. Be proactive in all respects concerning the board. Just because the board has authority in an area does not mean you should merely wait for the board to act and to instruct you. You are engaged in this work full time. You live and breathe it. That should lead to good ideas, deep insights, and refined analyses. The board depends on you for those benefits; don't bury your assets by excessive deference.

2. Never forget that the board prerogatives are theirs, not yours. The board, not you, has the ultimate authority for certain decisions and directions. You are a trusted adviser. That is a position of influence, not authority.

3. As CEO, and as a partner of the board, you should have great interest in getting the right people on the bus as board members. You should encourage and facilitate board self-evaluation and ensure that proper attention and lead time are provided for the nomination process. You can recommend processes, identify role models, suggest educational opportunities, and propose schedules that help the board fulfill this responsibility. That is part of your "consulting" role. The quality of your relationship with your board chair will be a major factor in your ability to advance these ideas.

4. Creating a skills and attributes grid to summarize the desired characteristics of board members and to identify how the board stacks up is not a job that can be done completely in committee. It requires staff work to prepare a good draft for review, comment, and completion. The key words here are "staff work" and "draft." Your role is to facilitate the work of the board and to engage them in the process. By doing so you provide them with a tool they can use and, through modification, come to own.

5. Advance the cultivation of new board members by focusing on building relationships when you are engaged in community activities. The process of building relationships gives you an ideal opportunity to assess readiness for board membership and to grow the sense of organizational affiliation among community leaders without usurping the board's role in the actual selection. This way, you increase the likelihood of success in member selection, which creates a win-win for you and the board.

APPLICATION GUIDELINES FOR THE BOARD

1. Embrace the CEO's activism on behalf of the board, but do not allow yourself to become lulled into a passive state, looking to the CEO to assume your responsibilities or to make decisions that are yours to make. Considering the CEO a trusted advisor does not mean suspending your own judgment.

2. Focus first on the mission of the organization and then on the results that are achieved by management and the medical staff. As not-for-profit board members, you are the trustees of the community's interests. Focusing on the mission will ensure that you do not get sidetracked into administrative work or responsibilities. Your passion for the mission will be a great attractor for the people you want on board. Focusing on outcomes will fulfill the responsibilities to the community you have as board members.

3. Look beyond the usual and obvious candidates for board positions. Identify people with backgrounds, skills, and perspectives that will enrich your board. Do not limit the board, the CEO, and the organization by narrow choices. Stretch them instead by seeking candidates with a broad range of skills and experiences.

4. Assessing board skills can be a difficult process for the board and CEO in terms of objectivity about the abilities found or not found among the current members of the board. Both may avoid making assessments that hint of criticism or deficiency. As board members, you should signal your willingness to be objective about yourselves as individuals and as a group. (See Chapter 7, "Board Appraisal and Development.")

5. The CEO is not the only one who should actively cultivate potential board members. You should understand this as one of your inherent responsibilities. You are in an excellent position to recruit by being open and positive about the health system and your experiences as board members. It is a virtuous cycle. Good people attract more good people.

REFERENCE

Collins, J. 2001. *Good to Great.* New York: HarperCollins.

CHAPTER 2

PHYSICIANS ON BOARDS

My first senior management meetings as vice president of a hospital were filled with a tension I hadn't expected. The neurosurgeons were urging all other surgeons to stop scheduling elective procedures as a protest against rising malpractice insurance rates. This threatened both our service mission and our financial stability. Coming to terms with this challenge would have been difficult under any circumstances. What made it even tougher, however, was that one of the protest leaders also served as president of the medical staff. As such, he attended our board meetings and senior management meetings as a non-voting medical staff representative.

Given the nature of the immediate threat, I could not understand why the board and CEO accepted this practice. The proposed slow-down would result in severely lower volumes and revenues. As VP for human resources, I had to design a contingency plan to cut pay and/or hours of staff throughout the hospital, from top to bottom. I was angry with the president of the medical staff, and I had difficulty containing my feelings in meetings where he was involved.

At the eleventh hour, the governor and the state legislature crafted a compromise solution, and the crisis passed. The surgeons did not interrupt any of their services, and my contingency plan was not activated. The president of the medical staff went on to perform in that role with distinction, just as he had done in the operating room. He was later elected to the board in his own right. He chaired the professional practice committee and became a close adviser to the CEO. Ultimately, he came to be one of the "wise old dogs" of the medical staff and an intelligent and knowledgeable voice of reason on the board to whom others turned for insight and perspective. He aligned himself with progressive efforts to improve hospital and physician performance.

I became CEO after he had retired from practice and moved from the community. I missed the opportunity to work closely with him, but we got together when he was in town to share a cup of coffee and talk about the changing state of affairs in healthcare. Like my predecessors, I found him to be committed to healthcare and willing to speak his mind even when his views departed from the mainstream. His outspokenness, which I had initially reacted against, proved in the long run to be one of his traits I most admired and valued. His clinical experience and reputation lent him credibility that he backed up with thoughtful analysis and good judgment. His example taught me about the very special contributions a physician can make to both board and management deliberations in healthcare.

BENEFITS OF PHYSICIANS AS BOARD MEMBERS

Physicians add a special dimension to healthcare boards. In contrast to many board members who feel intimidated by the specialized knowledge required in healthcare, physicians are in their element. For most of them, intensive exposure to hospitals began by their third year of medical school and continued throughout their internship and residency training. By the time they are under consideration for board membership, most physicians have intimate knowledge of healthcare language and processes—at least in their areas of specialization. The requirements of healthcare board membership that are most alien to lay board members fit squarely within a physician's comfort zone, so they are able to contribute to board effectiveness in several important ways.

Many board members are surprised to learn as part of their orientation that the law considers them to possess the final accountability for the quality of care in their organizations. They exercise this power through medical staff credentialing and through the performance improvement process. Without trusted and competent physician guides and partners, many lay board members would flounder in these areas. Without physician members, many boards would not possess the necessary knowledge to exercise judgment independent of management when confronting clinical quality issues.

Physician board members can also bring the voice of the patient into the boardroom. Because of their daily engagement with patients, they have more firsthand data and information about the realities of patient care than most of the non-physician board members and most of management. Physicians have a passion for patient care that ties them to the core purpose of the healthcare system.

Many physicians also advance organizational strategy because they are tuned in to innovations in medicine and technology—often more so than administration. By virtue of their knowledge and insights, they can add perspective to the considerations of the board regarding strategic and tactical options. Marketers of medical supplies and equipment target physicians through multiple channels, attempting to influence their purchase decisions. This presents a danger of unwise or unnecessary acquisitions but also guarantees a steady stream of information that many physicians can filter and apply on the organization's behalf.

Because of the obvious benefits physicians bring to their boards, many healthcare organizations specify a target percentage of board slots to be filled by physicians. They also add physicians to their boards for political and economic reasons. Physicians can make or break a hospital financially. In hospitals, it is essential that physicians as a group feel enfranchised and empowered. In the setup of American healthcare, patient care is fundamentally a partnership between physicians and the community as represented by the community's investment in the hospital as a place for physicians to care for patients.

POTENTIAL NEGATIVES OF PHYSICIAN BOARD MEMBERSHIP

Despite the obvious benefits, physicians on boards present special challenges to administration and to the rest of the board. Real or potential conflicts of interest often undermine the theoretical partnership between healthcare organizations and physicians. Indeed, conflicts are inherent both in the politics of healthcare and in the reimbursement system. For example, regulators attempt to use hospitals as an enforcement arm in overseeing the quality of physician care rather than doing so directly. In addition, payers reward hospitals and physicians in ways that often are directly contradictory, such as by negotiating a flat case rate with hospitals while paying physicians for each service provided. Moreover, through its anti-kickback regulations, the federal government has specifically ruled out some of the most practical and obvious opportunities for physician and healthcare organizations to reduce costs and increase revenue collaboratively and to share in the benefits. For example, government regulations prohibit most forms of gain-sharing where hospitals and physicians would split the savings derived from more efficient use of supplies. As a result, they often find themselves working at cross-purposes.

As physicians attempt to maintain or grow their income, the most attractive opportunities often put them into conflict with institutional interests. It is not unusual for physicians to resist the recruitment or credentialing of new physicians. What the hospital may see as added resources and new revenue streams, physicians may consider threats to their economic status quo and well-being.

Physicians and hospitals may also become direct competitors. Imagine the challenge for a physician who is a member of a group practice to also serve on a health system board. As each organization considers its financial situation and market options, the physician—who is privy to the confidential deliberations of each—must figure out how to balance conflicting loyalties and responsibilities. Some manage with impressive skill and judgment, but not all can do so.

TOWN HALL DEMOCRACY VERSUS REPRESENTATIONAL DEMOCRACY

Boards often invite physician leaders to join them to provide representation for physicians in governance. Although understandable, this motivation creates governance problems and also fails to achieve its aims. As in a New England town hall meeting, each physician reserves the right to speak for himself or herself. Many administrators have experienced attacks on their credibility by physicians who complain that actions were taken without physician input. These physicians do not consider elected medical staff leadership or physician board members to be speaking on their behalf: "You may have spoken to *those* doctors, but *we* weren't consulted."

This problem is compounded because the physicians on the board often do feel an obligation to speak as representatives of the medical staff at large, even while the medical staff judges such representation inadequate. Board members should not assume advocacy positions for subgroups, but physician board members—and often other board members—expect physicians to speak on behalf of physicians. That introduces unwarranted representational politics into board deliberations, without an offsetting benefit. Expecting a board member to represent an interest group violates the board principle of working on behalf of the best interests of the whole organization. Expecting physician board members to speak on behalf of physicians is not only wrong but also ineffective.

COACHING PHYSICIANS

This set of circumstances presents an ideal opportunity for a CEO who uses some of the approaches of a consultant to the board. By creating a bond with physician board members, the CEO can significantly advance the effectiveness of the board and the mission of the organization. Physicians often find themselves impatient and irritated with board processes. Things on the board do not work as they expect. They find themselves frustrated unless they receive timely, constructive, and gentle advice. A CEO who wants physician board members to succeed can provide private insights and suggest ways that physicians can work more effectively with their board colleagues.

Physicians have so many skills and such obvious understanding of patient care issues that it is easy for them and others to overlook glaring developmental needs associated with a lack of previous board experience. Without guidance and support, physicians may respond as many others do when thrown into unfamiliar situations with alien processes and uncertain rewards. They will criticize, withdraw, or become passive-aggressive.

A CEO "consultant" can help guide physician board members through the minefield of bureaucracy, to their mutual advantage. If physicians learn how to get things done through the give-and-take of group process where there is not necessarily a direct line to a solution, their impatience will not grow out of control. And if a CEO listens to physician board members the way a consultant listens to clients, he or she will gain new insights into organizational needs and opportunities. Consultants understand that their clients have firsthand experiences and complementary skills that will make the consultant's own performance even more impressive if he or she listens and learns well. CEOs should not miss this opportunity.

Table 2.1 Contrasts Between Managerial and Physician Orientations

Managers	Physicians
Organizational power derived from position	Professional power derived from knowledge
Develop processes	Give orders
Make rules for patient care	Break rules if necessary to meet patient needs
Agile and comfortable in bureaucratic settings	More comfortable in entrepreneurial environments
Accountable for revenues and expenses	Accountable for patient care and outcomes
Mistakes are part of learning	Errors can be fatal
Comfortable with representation	One person, one vote

Table 2.1 displays some characteristics that commonly differ between managers as a group and physicians as a group. A CEO with sensitivity to these contrasts can help both groups understand each other better and appreciate each other more.

APPLICATION GUIDELINES FOR THE CEO

1. Physician board members can provide an excellent reality check for your plans and programs. Be sure to listen to the facts and perspectives they offer, even when you question their intentions.

2. Do not assume your physician board members serve as representatives of physicians on your medical staff. Just because physician board members have had input does not mean other physicians will agree that medical staff issues have been adequately considered. You cannot substitute having a few physician board members for frequent and focused interactions with a broad cross-section of the medical staff.

3. Develop prospective physician board members. Seek out opportunities to put them into leadership roles or onto committees dealing with complex or controversial topics. Help them develop their skills and enhance their credibility as leaders. Do not undermine their legitimacy, however, by pushing them into roles as apologists for administration.

4. Be alert to potential conflicts of interest. If you identify such situations early, you will be in a position to have a healthy dialogue in advance with the affected physician. In addition to heading off conflicts or embarrassment, this may also prompt constructive discussions about areas for organizational growth and development. (See also the discussion on conflicts of interest in Chapter 9.)

5. Continue to coach physicians after they join the board. Provide opportunities for them to get further education on management, board, and healthcare topics. Help them broaden the scope of their contributions to board responsibilities. Encourage their involvement with committees that will prepare them for more comprehensive board participation and leadership.

APPLICATION GUIDELINES FOR THE BOARD

1. As is true for senior management, other board members should look to their physician colleagues for a reality check on management's plans and programs. Physician board members are generally supportive of management actions and proposals. If they are expressing reservations, be prepared to take a closer look.

2. Do not become overly dependent on physician board members in terms of the quality responsibilities of the board. Lay board members may not fully understand the clinical issues, but they can sometimes identify dynamics that insiders miss. In addition, physician board members can sometimes be

conflict-avoidant when dealing with the problems of their peers. Lay board members do not have the same burden of pre-existing professional and referral relationships.

3. Do not believe everything you hear. Physicians have an excellent vantage point from which to comment on healthcare operations. However, their individual roles do not necessarily provide them the benefit of the big picture. Listen, ask thoughtful and probing questions, and make your own judgments.

4. All board members have the potential for conflicts of interest—some more than others. A robust conflict policy, broadly understood and applied consistently, will enable the board to police itself. If the board deals reasonably and objectively with conflicts of interest, potential conflicts involving physicians will not become a source of discomfort, unacknowledged tensions, and hidden agendas.

5. Other board members have skills and experiences that many physicians may lack. For example, other board members may have more business education and business experience. Board members will find many of their physician colleagues eager to learn from them. They will contribute to the education of physicians if they explain the reasons for their opinions and offer supporting examples. A healthy dialogue based on mutual respect will help build an outstanding board.

CHAPTER 3

THE CHAIR AND THE EXECUTIVE COMMITTEE

FIRST AMONG EQUALS

GEORGE ORWELL'S *Animal Farm* proclaims, "All animals are equal, but some animals are more equal than others." In just 12 words, Orwell captured the frequent reality of unequal power and influence among the members of even the most democratically organized groups. Inequality of influence often exists within not-for-profit boards of trustees. In particular, the board chair and the executive committee generally have access to more information, operate closer to the center of power, and have more opportunities for input than do other members of the board. In some cases, bylaws confer on the executive committee the power to act in place of the board between board meetings.

The executive committee constitutes the leadership cadre of the board. If board succession planning works as it should, it is likely the committee can count among its number the next two or three board chairs.

When conflicts, controversies, or crises strike the organization, the board chair and other members of the executive committee get the first calls from the CEO. When the CEO needs a sounding board, the executive committee is commonly the first choice. Along with the CEO, the executive committee exercises the greatest control over which issues and proposals are brought to the full board. They often frame the recommendations for board consideration.

The board chair is an elite among elites. He or she develops a close working relationship with the CEO and is privy to confidential information and work in process. The chair sets or approves the board agenda, conducts the board meetings, and controls the flow of participation. With the CEO, the chair sets the tone for candor, caution, criticism, or conflict among the board members and with senior staff. The chair is the face of the board.

FIRST *WHO*, THEN *WHAT*

Jim Collins (2001, 42) teaches in *Good to Great*: "If you begin with 'who,' rather than 'what,' you can more easily adapt to a changing world. . . . [The right people] will be self-motivated by the inner drive . . . to be part of creating something great." Collins also recognizes the magnetic power of having the right people on board: They attract others like themselves to sign up for board service.

Leaders of the board should be members of the "in" group in more ways than one. Because they exercise so much power and have such an impact on performance, they should possess character and skills commensurate with the job. It would be easy for CEOs to generate long lists of desirable traits, like those found in their own job descriptions, such as walking on water and leaping tall buildings.

I have found, however, that a simple five-word list suffices as a starting point. I call these the five "ins." Board leaders should display *in*tegrity, *in*telligence, *in*sight, *in*tuition, and *in*fluence.

Integrity

Not-for-profit organizations and healthcare organizations should be mission-driven. However, as they grow in size, and as reimbursement becomes both lucrative and threatened, mission and purpose often slide to back-of-mind consideration. "No margin, no mission" is a truism, but it is also a cover for those who do not want to cloud pursuit of profit with questions of purpose. Along with the CEO, the chair and the executive committee apply value judgments to the work of the organization. There are many financial, political, and social pressures on healthcare leaders. It is easy to lose direction without leaders with integrity, guided by the organization's mission. In addition, integrity is a key ingredient in building trust among the members of the board and with the CEO.

Intelligence

Change and uncertainty demand intelligence from executives and boards. Little in healthcare works in a simple or straightforward way. Understanding the illogic of healthcare reimbursement requires simultaneous consideration of multiple factors and variables. Leaders must be able to learn quickly and remember facts and principles. A CEO who is trying to move the organization in new directions needs board leaders who get it. Board leaders who cannot readily process new information and perspectives limit the ability of the organization to respond to changing markets and new approaches to care.

Insight

One of the most important board skills is the ability to see beneath the surface and beyond the current situation. This requires more than just general intelligence. Insight is the ability to detect trends or hidden currents. Insight asks the question, "What is changing, and what does it mean?" Insight also asks, "Why?" "Why were the results different from what we expected?" "Why was the reaction to the proposal so strong?" Board leaders with insight challenge and comfort a CEO. They do not settle for superficial answers. They help the CEO see troubling situations or emerging issues with greater clarity.

Intuition

A couple of steps beyond insight, intuition is understanding something before you know why you know it. Like insight, intuition derives from experience, especially experience a leader has carefully attended to and reflected on.

Because bias sometimes masquerades as intuition, intuitions need to be shared and debated. CEOs who can openly discuss intuitions with their boards will be better positioned to recognize new possibilities and problems. They can raise issues for consideration before sufficient evidence is available to develop conclusions deductively. CEOs and board leaders who engage in active and candid dialogue can test and sharpen their intuitive skills for the benefit of the organization.

Influence

The most effective board leaders are those who can influence others without the direct exercise of power. Such leaders are persuasive, either as a matter of style or as a matter of stature. Others look to them for ideas, comments, or confirmation. Some board leaders play down their influence to boost participation and feelings of collaboration. They should not, however, ignore or misperceive group dynamics. Groups do not come to conclusions or make decisions easily. A leader who can use influence judiciously can build strength, confidence, and mutual regard within the board as it deals with challenging issues.

Moreover, the organization and the CEO need allies in the community. Board members with influence enhance the stature of the organization and can help ease the way for new initiatives. A CEO and influential board members can gain access to funders, decision makers, regulators, and legislators in a way that can be difficult for a CEO alone to manage.

GROOMING OFFICERS

Fewer healthcare organizations operate without term limits than was true a decade ago, before the increased scrutiny of for-profit and not-for-profit boards. This makes grooming officers even more of a challenge. Potential officers need to be identified early in their first term, or service limits may come into play before they have had the opportunity to exercise formal board leadership. CEOs should work with their board chairs to spot talent.

Just as the CEO looks for inquisitiveness and intelligence to identify prospective board members, so should the CEO and board chair stay alert to signs of talent and commitment among new members. It usually takes a year or two for a board member to get up to speed because of the new language, finances, regulations, and organizational oddities of healthcare. Nevertheless, potential leaders emerge during this time. The CEO should test the waters with good prospects before the end of their second year. In many cases, opportunities to do so present themselves when emerging leaders seek out the CEO to ask questions, check their understanding, or gain additional insights. Patient and encouraging responses often lead to more dialogue and strengthen the board member's commitment to the organization. The CEO and the chair can suggest specific learning opportunities. If there are conferences or audio programs, they can extend personal invitations to board members showing leadership aptitude.

Under ideal circumstances, the CEO, the chair, and the governance committee will nominate prospective board officers to committee leadership posts by their third or fourth year on the board. By then, emerging leaders will have gained credibility with their peers and will have sufficient understanding of organizational issues to take on leadership positions.

In many organizations, chairing a standing committee qualifies the chair for membership on the executive committee. This opens three more important developmental opportunities. First, most CEOs use the executive committee as a sounding board. This will help draw prospective officers into the complexities, uncertainties, and strategies of the organization. Moreover, it exposes them more deeply to the work of all the functional committees. Finally, by serving as leaders, they begin to self-identify as leaders. This becomes a mutually reinforcing positive cycle.

DEVELOPING RELATIONSHIPS

A CEO who wants strong board leadership will seek to build mutual trust, confidence, and respect. This is so important for the board as a whole that Chapter 10 is devoted to this topic.

The chair and the executive committee should create bonds that enable members to challenge and test each other without causing hard feelings or engendering defensiveness. People who have personal and professional regard for each other can manage difficult situations and differences of opinion without taking them personally.

The CEO and the chair need to look beyond the business at hand and attend to their own relationship and the relationships among all the members of the executive committee. A savvy CEO will supplement work sessions with incidental and planned social interaction. Spending time to get to know each other personally is a building block of board strength, not a diversion of board energy. Personal regard and trust do more to hold people together than roles or titles alone.

If the relationship between the CEO and the chair breaks down, however, the entire organization may be affected. Clashing personalities, different visions for the organization, or a misunderstanding of their respective roles may lead to tests of will, disharmony, and dysfunction. In those circumstances, CEOs and chairs may find it helpful to seek outside help. This is one instance where the model of a CEO as an internal consultant may be ineffective. An external consultant who can work with both parties objectively can defuse tensions and provide a starting point for attitude and behavior change. Conflicts between the CEO and the chair cost the organization money, time, momentum, and spirit. Some of these situations do resolve themselves with time, but dealing with them proactively is more effective. Getting outside help is a constructive response to this type of problem.

APPLICATION GUIDELINES FOR THE CEO

1. The responsibilities of the board chair weigh heavily on many who take the role. You do both of yourselves a favor when you mentor your "boss." Providing support and affirmation reduces stress, especially early on. Never doubt that the selection of the board chair is critical. Do not settle for compromises. Be aware that if you and the chair do not groom upcoming leaders, the board's choices for future leadership may be limited.

2. You and the chair set the tone for the board in terms of style and values. This is a long, cumulative process, but progress can be undone easily, and repairs are difficult.

3. Conflict can be constructive, especially if you and your board leaders are trying to develop your intuition and insight. Work

with your chair and executive committee so that everyone feels comfortable testing ideas before they are fully formed.

4. Reach out to new board members. Even if they do not know it, they are auditioning for board leadership positions. You want to assess their aptitudes and inclinations for leading. Enlist your chair and executive committee, and share your assessments with them.

5. Attend to the mix of styles, backgrounds, and experiences of the members of the executive committee. You want members who can work together and who rank high on the five "ins." However, you also need individuals with different points of view and temperaments who can balance and stretch each other and you.

APPLICATION GUIDELINES FOR THE BOARD

1. Board leadership brings many responsibilities. Do not select people for leadership and then abandon them. Volunteer to help; do not delegate up.

2. In some groups, leadership positions are rotated among all members. Sometimes they wish to ensure that no one feels excluded. In other cases, board leadership selection resembles a game of musical chairs where each person eventually gets stuck with the job. Avoid this temptation. It will not serve you, the organization, or the CEO well.

3. If you demand perfection, penalize mistakes, or scoff at ideas, you will never achieve the openness of discussion that leads to genuine insights. Give yourself and your CEO permission to stretch in the idea department. You are likely to uncover hidden talents on the board if you do.

4. With stronger attention to term limits, board succession is more difficult to choreograph. Help newcomers get up to

speed. If you spot talent, encourage and support deeper involvement.

5. Look for opportunities where you can help the CEO make connections in the community. Board members who include the CEO and each other in business, civic, and social activities broaden and strengthen the reach of the organization in the community.

REFERENCE

Collins, J. 2001. *Good to Great.* New York: HarperCollins.

CHAPTER 4

CEO BOARD PARTICIPATION, SUCCESSION PLANNING, AND SELECTION

YOU CAN FIND almost anything on the Internet. You can access information, comparison shop, find a new house, get replacement parts for an appliance, even buy Finnish cinnamon toast from a family bakery in northern Michigan. You can qualify for free shipping, avoid sales taxes, and buy at deeply discounted prices. But you can't get a CEO.

Wouldn't boards love to be able to scan through hundreds of CEO choices, sorted by cost, popularity, and user ratings? Instead, they must do it the old-fashioned way: through word of mouth and trial and error. Boards may hire consultants to help, but although search firms have experience and data banks, they work essentially the same way.

Healthcare bylaws often designate the CEO a voting member of the board. Even without voting membership, however, the CEO attends board meetings, sets agendas, and coordinates board activities. Thus, selecting a CEO, voting member or not, means inviting a new and influential person into the existing board mixture.

CEOS AS BOARD MEMBERS: PROS AND CONS

Should CEOs be voting members of their boards? Although academics might debate this, it often seems more a matter of tradition than a conscious decision. Sometimes a CEO candidate will insist on a commitment of board membership before accepting an offer, but often the issue of board membership goes unnoticed and unremarked. It shouldn't. Boards should consider this option, and the CEO as consultant should help—even if there is a potential conflict of interest.

Table 4.1 lists some of the factors a board should consider when deciding whether or not a CEO should be a voting member of the board.

It is difficult for CEOs to completely put aside personal feelings when consulting with their boards about this issue. In fact, they shouldn't, because CEO satisfaction is a relevant factor. However, consideration of how these issues and others like them play out in the board and the organization is more important.

For example, a history of troubled board and CEO relations might tempt the board to exclude the CEO from membership. However, CEO board membership may be most helpful in a case like this. Likewise, if the organization is in building mode, CEO board membership may support development. On the other hand, if the board has been lax in fulfilling its responsibilities or has not stepped up to challenges, CEO membership may compound the problem. How these factors play out is a function of local history and considerations, but it should be evaluated consciously, at least at the time of transition.

SETTING EXPECTATIONS

If the CEO is included on the board, what are the appropriate expectations for how the CEO will act? The question illuminates the issue: The CEO is not just like any other board member. As a

Table 4.1 Considerations Related to CEO Membership on Not-for-Profit Boards

CEO **Should Be** a Board Member	CEO **Should NOT Be** a Board Member
• Supports equality of status	• The board hires, evaluates, and compensates the CEO
• Lessens "us" vs. "them" (management vs. board)	• It is unnecessary as the CEO already has the clout of chief executive
• Increases accountability for decisions	• Potential conflicts of interest
• Makes exclusion from board processes more difficult	• CEO membership:
• May improve communications between boards in multi-board systems	▪ May lessen the independence of the board—actual or perceived
• Adds status when needed in discussions with potential external organizational partners	▪ May muddle the respective responsibilities of board and management
• Occasionally facilitates quorums, especially in committees	▪ May lessen participation by others
	▪ May decrease credibility of board as community based

full-time, paid employee with executive authority, the CEO generally possesses greater industry and organizational knowledge. That expertise should not translate into a dominant role in board discussions, however; that would undermine the very foundation of a governing board.

Nevertheless, in many healthcare board meetings the CEO takes the lead role on each agenda item. Presentations take precedence over discussion. Such dynamics encourage board members to become passive observers rather than leaders. Figure 4.1 describes the relationship between CEO activity and board passivity. As can be seen, this is a classic S-curve. As the level of CEO participation increases, the level of board activity rapidly decreases. This doesn't mean CEOs cannot participate in

Figure 4.1 Impact of Increasing CEO Participation on Level of Board Activity

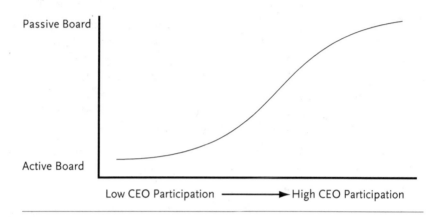

board meetings, but the negative consequences multiply quickly past a minimal level of participation.

Therefore, CEOs who wish to have active boards need to calibrate their own participation carefully. This can be difficult because boards look to CEOs to present timely and vital information. They want CEOs to respond knowledgeably to inquiries. Boards recognize their own lack of expertise and depend on CEOs to provide background and context. All of this tempts CEOs to overparticipate. Before they realize it, they have enabled boards to move from active to passive.

The CEO as consultant should work with the board chair and executive committee or with the governance committee to establish expectations for the CEO's role as a board member. Ideally, this will create a shared understanding that the CEO's role as a presenter will normally not exceed a targeted threshold (e.g., 20 percent of a board meeting). Moreover, the chair and the CEO will encourage multilateral discussions around the board table rather than serial dialogues between the CEO and other board members in turn. The CEO's goal should be to create a board process where all members of the board feel shared responsibility for the success of the meeting.

DIRECT ROLE IN SUCCESSION PLANNING

The CEO and the board share responsibility for succession planning. In theory, this ranks as one of their most important responsibilities, but in practice it often lags behind more immediate duties. Many boards and CEOs actually avoid the discussion. The topic itself seems to imply disloyalty, so if discussed at all, it is cloaked in the language of "if the CEO happened to be hit by a truck tomorrow...."

There is no need to be so delicate. Reframe the task as *developmental* planning rather than *replacement* planning. A CEO should be engaged in developmental planning with subordinates even if he or she has no intentions of leaving within the foreseeable future. The following questions apply as the CEO reviews each direct report or other future leaders:

- Which of this executive's strengths in his or her current position can be built on?
- What gaps in this person's experience should be addressed?
- What additional opportunities or responsibilities will provide the best learning experiences for this executive?
- How do this person's background, style, and skills match the organization's present and future needs?
- How much capacity for additional growth does this person appear to possess?
- Are there factors that rule out further advancement for this executive?
- Does this person demonstrate potential to lead the organization in the future?
- What should the CEO do next to help prepare this individual

to achieve greater personal success and contribute more to the advancement of the organization?

CEOs who complete these reviews are well prepared to discuss succession with their boards because planning for succession is fundamentally about developing leadership talent within organizations. Annual reviews with board leadership help ensure that both parties are fulfilling their obligations regarding the identification and preparation of future leaders. The transition to specific succession planning is easier and less threatening for both the CEO and the board once the CEO, as consultant, has laid the foundation.

INDIRECT ROLE IN SELECTION

The recommendation to act like a consultant to the board runs into complications when it comes to the board's responsibility for CEO selection. Given the significant potential for conflicts of interest (e.g., an out-going CEO's desire to be respected and warmly remembered versus an organization's need to chart a new path), it takes great personal discipline and maturity for a CEO to be an unbiased consultant.

Unless there is a clear internal candidate for succession, boards generally form committees to guide the process and coordinate the search and interviews. Many healthcare organizations use search consultants to assist with CEO selection. CEOs should provide space and freedom of movement to the board, the committee, and the search consultant. However, it would be a mistake for CEOs to abdicate all responsibility in the process. CEOs should ensure that certain materials are available for board and consultant review:

- A current job description
- An assessment of current organizational performance against the annual budget and the long-term strategic plan
- The most recent developmental assessments of internal

organizational leaders along with appropriate updates
- A forecast of issues and opportunities over the next 24–48 months
- A personal assessment of the CEO–board relationship and recommendations for changes

CEOs normally develop a positive sense of ownership of their organizations. They find it difficult to be hands-off when it comes to such an important process and decision. CEOs and board chairs should construct an approach that will keep the CEO informed and provide a route for sharing input or concerns. However, this agreement should keep the CEO out of direct participation in selection discussions or other activities where he or she might unduly influence other board members. CEO transitions provide the opportunity for course correction, but direct CEO participation reduces the likelihood that discussions will take place as they should. Therefore, even if the out-going CEO is a board member, he or she should not participate in the executive sessions when the board discusses the selection process. The board chair should maintain an active dialogue with the CEO about this process, however.

APPLICATION GUIDELINES FOR THE CEO

1. If you are not a board member and if board membership is appropriate in your organizational context, do not hesitate to raise the issue.
2. It is in your and the organization's best interest to establish peer relationships with the board, increase the sense of shared accountability, and minimize barriers between you and the board.
3. CEOs who dominate board meetings, particularly by overdoing presentations, enable the board to evade its responsibilities. Do not be an enabler.
4. Planning for succession is theoretically the board's

responsibility, but in practice, you are much better positioned to take the lead. You can assess potential successors, identify individual needs and opportunities, review this with the board and the executives themselves, and put developmental plans into action. The CEO of General Electric is reported to spend more than 10 percent of his time on leadership development. What about you?

5. Unless you have done an exceptional job of internal development, you will rarely have the opportunity to select your own successor. That does not mean, however, that you should keep your influence entirely out of the process. Respect the board's authority, but facilitate the process by providing specific, targeted information and insights. You may be in a better position than anyone else to provide this information and insight.

APPLICATION GUIDELINES FOR THE BOARD

1. "This is the way we have always done it" is not a sufficient reason to include or not include your CEO on your board.

2. If you are uncertain whether your CEO has the skills, stature, personality, or other qualifications for the board, then he or she is not likely to have the qualities needed to be CEO, either.

3. Increase the vitality of board meetings by interacting directly with other board members in discussion: Ask questions, build on comments, support good ideas, raise alternatives, and challenge perceptions. This helps the CEO maintain an appropriate activity level in board meetings.

4. Formalize the succession planning process to ensure the board and CEO attend to it and discuss it at least annually. Talent development is one of those important but usually not urgent activities that easily get pushed aside. See also Chapter 8.

5. As much as you may respect your out-going CEO, remember that CEO transition presents a superb opportunity for course correction and revitalization. This is natural. Do not let your regard for the incumbent cause you to shortchange the organization.

SECTION II

WHAT?

CHAPTER 5

DEFINING PURPOSE AND SETTING DIRECTION

YEARS AGO, I consulted with a high-tech start-up company that exemplified the challenge of defining purpose. It was a wholly owned subsidiary of a consortium of companies, and it existed to serve the technology needs of the owners. But this left its direction undefined. I began a team-building workshop by organizing top management into teams to review their mission and vision. Usually new teams struggle with reconciling different perspectives, but these teams didn't. I discovered as I reviewed their output that each team simply incorporated individual views by stringing them together. This reflected the way the organization had skipped past the difficult work of developing a focus. We altered the intended agenda and devoted significant time to this issue. Without a shared understanding of mission and vision, the organization could not capitalize on its talent and financial resources. Many healthcare and other not-for-profit organizations face the same challenge.

ELEVATING COMMUNITY STEWARDSHIP

In *The Art of Getting Your Own Sweet Way,* Phillip Crosby (1981, 9) writes, "The primary concern of management is survival." He contends that understanding this motivation would help others work with managers more successfully. Crosby was not being cynical, and I have taken the same posture in using his principle over the years to better understand organizational behavior.

For example, Crosby's principle came into play when I consulted on the potential merger of two not-for-profit community organizations whose target clients and funders overlapped considerably. Although the two organizations took different approaches to their service offerings, the funders had decided they could no longer support the competition between them. I investigated the factors that had doomed previous merger discussions, and discovered that the boards of both organizations had great loyalty toward their respective CEOs. A combined organization would only need one. The prospective merger could not proceed until the boards came to terms with this issue. From the outside, the community benefit objective was clear, but to those inside, the conflict between community benefit and personal loyalty presented more difficulty. Some of the board members behaved as if their CEO's employment security was the primary purpose of the organization.

When its purpose gets blurry, an organization tends to take its very existence as its central purpose. As Crosby puts it, "The primary concern . . . is survival."

In not-for-profit healthcare, boards are the stewards of an important community resource. Survival is not a trivial concern. Healthcare organizations must generate surpluses to continue operation. They face the multiple pressures of free enterprise and public policy and regulation. Maintaining a sense of purpose becomes difficult. Healthcare boards have a responsibility to their communities, but they can lose their sense of direction. CEOs can serve their boards, their communities, and their organizations well by helping their boards stay focused on purpose and mission.

CREATING A UNIQUE MISSION AND VISION

Do an Internet search for the missions and visions of healthcare organizations and you will find striking similarities among organizations and from town to town. You will read phrases such as these:

- "to advance the health and well-being of the communities of ___"
- "committed to promoting, improving, and enhancing the health and well-being of the community we serve"
- "to provide compassionate, accessible, high-quality, cost-effective healthcare to the community"
- "care for the people of our community by providing advanced and compassionate healthcare of superior quality and value"

These phrases are echoed by hundreds of hospitals around the country. What, if anything, makes each mission statement unique?

In *Competing for the Future*, Hamel and Prahalad (1994, 22) argue that to be a leader in its field, an organization must be different from its competitors. Just being better is not enough. As they say: "The goal is not simply to benchmark a competitor's products and processes and imitate its methods, but to develop an independent point of view about tomorrow's opportunities and how to exploit them." Healthcare organizations, however, are often mired in a game of follow-the-leader. Many large consulting organizations seem to make their living selling the same solutions over and over again to health systems across the country. Given the relatively decentralized nature of the industry, it is not surprising that benchmarking and adopting best practices are so common. This is not a bad thing. These approaches help raise the overall performance of healthcare providers. However, benchmarking and best practices fundamentally create good followers, not good leaders. CEOs and boards should identify opportunities to be unique in their markets. They should add value beyond the ordinary expectations for healthcare organizations.

VALUES IN PRINCIPLE VERSUS VALUES IN ACTION

Richard Bernstein (1971) draws a distinction between values in principle—those you profess—and values in action—those that actually guide your behavior. CEOs and boards should understand this distinction and identify values that will truly guide the work of their organizations.

Patrick Lencioni (2002, 114) has taken this same idea and describes values in a way that most leaders will be able to recognize. He places values into four categories:

1. **Core values**: "the deeply ingrained principles that guide all of a company's actions"
2. **Aspirational values**: "those that a company needs to succeed in the future but currently lacks"
3. **Permission-to-play values**: those that "simply reflect the minimal social and behavioral standards required of any employee"
4. **Accidental values**: those that "reflect the common interests or personalities of the organization's employees" but may not be related to purpose or success

To these, I have added a fifth:

5. **Counterfeit values**: those an organization claims but does not practice

If someone watched you or your organization in action, would that observer be able to identify your professed principles and values? If not, it is likely that you or your organization are not living your values. The Enron Corporation had an extraordinary set of written values. However, if you had observed the company in action you would never have guessed what those values were. They were counterfeit values.

Does your organization have distinctive, core values that make you who you are? Or are your values the worthy but non-distinctive permission-to-play values Lencioni described? Alternatively, do you declare values that are lofty but not accurately descriptive of your organization? Do you profess certain values, but reward others? These are questions boards should ask and answer.

THE STRATEGIC PLAN

The CEO and board pull together the mission, vision, values, environmental assessment, and competitive business case for the organization in the strategic plan. What is the organization's value proposition? What does it offer the community in return for support and patronage?

Unfortunately, boards often take a passive role in this process. As Chait, Ryan, and Taylor (2005, 54–55) note in *Governance as Leadership*, "The first and natural inclination of trustees is to do strategy the old way, much as boards do finance, facilities, and programs. Just as boards required and reviewed budgets, boards now expect to approve plans and monitor implementation. . . . Consistent with the view that organizational leaders bear responsibility for crafting strategy, trustees generally accept the substance of the plan with only minor modifications."

They suggest a different approach: "if an organization's strategy rests on new concepts and reconsidered value propositions, . . . a board must do more than mandate and monitor a plan. The role of the board shifts, in a way, from brawn to brains, from the power of the board's oversight . . . to the power of the board's ideas" (Chait, Ryan, and Taylor 2005, 65).

In this model, the CEO creates strategy *with* the board rather than *for* the board. Likewise, the board works *with* management to establish the basic direction and frame of reference for the plan rather than delegate those tasks *to* management. What the board does is work with the CEO to articulate a shared vision for the organization. It thus sharpens the focus for organizational investment and actions. It ensures management acts in the best interests of the owners (which for most healthcare organizations is the community). The strategic plan guides the development and implementation of annual operating plans and budgets. By operating at the 30,000-foot level rather than on the ground, the board can maintain a broader view, recognize patterns better, and see further ahead than managers and staff who must also be concerned with day-to-day activities.

APPLICATION GUIDELINES FOR THE CEO

1. It is easy to avoid difficult choices by trying to do a little of everything. This temptation affects both executives and boards. You need to help the board come to terms with this.

2. Passion drives excellence. Boards can lose their sense of passion and mission because they are so far from the organization's actual service delivery. When you help the board stay focused on purpose, you help sustain their passion and commitment. When you focus only on survival, the organization settles for mediocrity rather than striving for excellence.

3. Benchmarking and employing best practices are useful disciplines intended to help you serve your communities. They are necessary, but they are not sufficient to produce a great healthcare organization.

4. Great organizations usually rely on core, noneconomic values to weather crises. You can help your organization develop strong, reliable values by publicly holding yourself and others

accountable for compliance with your values and by inviting them to do the same.

5. Design your strategic planning process with meaningful board participation in mind. Include the board right from the start to engage their imagination and intelligence. Chait, Ryan, and Taylor (2005) provide helpful suggestions in this regard.

APPLICATION GUIDELINES FOR THE BOARD

1. As you define purpose, don't let loyalty to your CEO and staff take precedence over your obligation to the community and the mission of the organization.

2. Some healthcare organizations consider their community benefit a *given*. However, ordinary business pressures can cause not-for-profit organizations to drift from their missions. Do not allow mission to be merely a perfunctory, annual discussion in your organization.

3. Help the CEO understand the desires and values of the community in a more intimate way by sharing your understanding of them and by offering alternative perspectives on community needs and preferences.

4. Do not allow the review of organizational values to become a routine exercise. Do not allow values statements to "simply reflect the minimal social and behavioral standards required of any employee" (Lencioni 2002, 114). Help strengthen the organization by unearthing and articulating its core values.

5. Many boards defer to management in the articulation of the mission, vision, values, and strategy of the organization. Do not defer. Do not dominate. Be a partner. Collaborate.

REFERENCES

Bernstein, R. 1971. *Praxis and Action: Contemporary Philosophies of Human Activity*. Philadelphia: University of Pennsylvania Press.

Chait, R. P., W. P. Ryan, and B. P. Taylor. 2005. *Governance as Leadership: Reframing the Work of Nonprofit Boards*. Hoboken, NJ: John Wiley & Sons.

Crosby, P. 1981. *The Art of Getting Your Own Sweet Way*. New York: McGraw-Hill.

Hamel, G., and C. K. Prahalad. 1994. *Competing for the Future*. Boston: Harvard Business School Press.

Lencioni, P. 2002. "Make Your Values Mean Something." *Harvard Business Review* 80 (July): 113–117.

CHAPTER 6

MEASUREMENT: ESTABLISHING AND MAINTAINING STANDARDS

I ASKED A colleague, a senior executive in a high-tech firm, the secret to his company's soaring operational and financial results. "Breakthrough objectives," he said. His CEO had set targets so far above the ordinary that they forced the management team to abandon their usual methods and completely rethink how they went about their business. The CEO used these goals to raise company aspirations and redefine what was acceptable.

In healthcare, the CEO and the board share responsibility for establishing and maintaining standards. Chait, Ryan, and Taylor (2005) classify board work as *fiduciary* (concerned with the stewardship of tangible assets), *strategic* (concerned with performance in a changing environment), or *generative* (concerned with judgments about the meaning and purpose of the organization's work). However you conceive of a board's responsibilities, establishing and maintaining standards—through measurement—is key among them.

INTERNAL MEASUREMENT AND REPORTING

Measurement can alter goals and expectations, but it can also be a reality check. My experiences as a CEO and as a board member taught me that we often assumed a higher level of performance than careful measurement supported. Before we began rigorously monitoring patient satisfaction, overall quality, and safety, we estimated our performance at well above average, on the basis of our good intentions and level of effort. But when we measured ourselves with standardized tools, we identified significant service and quality gaps that compromised our overall performance. Some were easy to correct while others required sustained focus, but few would have been addressed as tenaciously or diligently without measurements to point the way.

I worked with a CEO who understood the way measurement benefited her and her organization. She devised a short, balanced scorecard for her organization and a comparable, parallel one for herself. She reviewed these with her board as part of her operating plan and annual performance objectives and made modifications based on the review. She included fewer than a dozen measures on each scorecard, with the ability to obtain more detailed measurements when necessary. She reported regularly on both. Although it was not always comfortable, she didn't back down or make excuses for unexpected outcomes.

As a result, she was able to consolidate gains, pinpoint problem areas early, and implement corrective action when needed. She operates in the difficult area of long-term care. Positive results are often fleeting, so she can never get complacent or rest on prior accomplishments. Nevertheless, despite setbacks, she has been able to garner state and national awards for quality and service.

No one, to my knowledge, has written better on this topic than Robert Kaplan and David Norton. Their three books—*The Balanced Scorecard* (1996), *The Strategy-Focused Organization* (2001), and *Strategy Maps* (2004)—describe the use of measurement to refine and focus organizational strategy. Two themes run through all three books with increasing clarity:

1. Organizations should not rely solely on financial measures to judge performance; they should also include operational and customer-focused measures.

2. The measures managers track should reflect their theory of the business. What measurable operational improvements lead to what customer outcomes, producing what financial results?

When executives use measurement this way, it moves from a bureaucratic paperwork exercise to an essential tool for defining strategy and marshalling resources to implement that strategy. And, of course, it enables managers to self-correct when performance does not match intentions.

Here are five basic principles for internal measurement for CEOs:

1. Work with your board to decide what measures to use and the targets for each. Do this prospectively rather than retrospectively.
2. Choose a small number of measures that reflect your theory of the business, as described in detail by Kaplan and Norton (2004).
3. Identify and commit to the measures so your employees and your board know what your key indicators of success are.
4. Monitor and report regularly and candidly, including trends over time, and require other managers to do the same at their organizational levels.
5. If properly chosen, these measures should direct day-to-day and longer-term actions. If not, you must determine whether you are using the wrong measures or focusing your efforts on the wrong factors.

EXTERNAL MEASUREMENT AND PERFORMANCE REPORTING

My brother-in-law, who lives in another state, called me for advice when he needed to be hospitalized. I was not personally familiar with the hospitals in his area, so I logged onto the

Internet to search publicly available report cards. I was 15 or 20 minutes into the process when I suddenly stopped and slapped myself like the actors do in the V8 commercials.

I had made a fundamental error. I knew that the public reporting available for the hospitals with which I was familiar had only a chance correlation with the real facts as I understood them. I could point to specific errors in reporting and to research that cast doubt on the overall accuracy and usefulness of such data. Nevertheless, I had done just what many other reasonable people would do in the absence of direct, reliable information: I turned to the Internet.

Healthcare organizations, their CEOs, and their boards need to catch up with this rapidly changing dynamic. Healthcare has always been a primarily local business with referrals based largely on reputation and word of mouth. I doubt that will ever change completely, but the Internet is fundamentally changing communications and purchasing behaviors across many areas of daily living. There is no reason to expect healthcare to be immune.

Public reporting creates six challenges CEOs and boards must address:

1. Different groups, each with different priorities and different levels of commitment to data integrity, are creating report cards.
2. The data used are often inconsistent among reporting groups.
3. There is no effective tool that satisfactorily equalizes results among different types of healthcare organizations.
4. Data submitted by providers are often not cross-validated, so data from different providers may not be comparable.
5. Some reports are generated from data collected for entirely different purposes, and some require new data collection, adding to overhead burdens.

6. Most data are out of date by the time they are accessible by the public, so reports will not reflect improvements or problems that have occurred since the data were originally generated.

The CEO consulting with the board will want to:

- educate the board on publicly available scorecards;
- identify those with the most credibility and impact, such as government reports on core measures;
- produce comparisons with competitors;
- identify meaningful strengths and shortcomings relative to agreed-on standards;
- map the relationship between the external measures and the reports routinely provided to the board; and
- discuss strategies for improving real organizational performance and organizational appearance on report cards, as the two may not be equivalent.

VARIANCE FROM STANDARDS

Managing variance from standards is a fundamental principle of general management and quality management. Quality guru W. E. Deming preaches the minimization of variation as the key to improving quality (Walton 1986), noting that top management must also identify and understand the causes for variation. However, Deming also recognizes that not everything important can be measured. Thus, one of the greatest proponents of statistical process control also advocates the use of judgment.

I recommend a three-step approach to variation derived from research on memory:

1. To manage variance, you need to *become aware* of variance. You cannot do this without maintaining routine measurement practices.
2. You must *pay attention* to variance. Implement a process to ensure systematic reviews of key organizational measures.
3. You must *put the measures in context.* Use a balanced scorecard or strategy map that relates your measures to your theory of the business.

In the language of memory research, this would constitute something memorable. In the language of management, it would constitute something important and controllable.

MEASUREMENT CAUTIONS

In the movie *Chicago*, attorney Billy Flynn did a soft-shoe routine and advised his prospective client, Roxie Hart, to "Give 'em the old Razzle Dazzle." Roxie stood accused of murder, but when I first heard the lyrics, my mind jumped immediately to some of the people I have watched over the years presenting reports loaded with numbers, tables, and charts. When people use statistics, make sure that they are not trying to "razzle dazzle" you.

In 1954, Darrell Huff wrote a deceptively simple little book intended as a cautionary tale, *How to Lie with Statistics*. It still sells well. In the introduction, he notes: "Averages and relationships and trends and graphs are not always what they seem. There may be more in them than meets the eye, and there may be a good deal less. The secret language of statistics . . . is employed to sensationalize, inflate, confuse, and oversimplify" (Huff 1993, 8).

So it can be with dashboards, balanced scorecards, and other tools executives use to measure and track objectives for performance improvement and reporting to the board. These tools can improve organizational effectiveness, but they can also give a misleading appearance of progress. This is especially true:

- if there is a large number of measures,
- if they are chosen retrospectively rather than prospectively, or
- if there is little or no understanding of the underlying activities that produce the measures.

If any of these conditions is true of measures presented for your review, be wary. Convincing explanations can be created for correlations that are actually random. Spurious "statistically significant" results are easily obtained from a large sample of results. (For example, given 100 measurements, it is likely that 5 will be significant at the 0.05 level by chance alone.) Finally, the terms *statistically significant* and *meaningful* are not equivalent. In statistics, significance is an assessment of whether or not a given observation is likely to have occurred by chance, not an assessment of its practical use. Good statisticians are careful with numbers. Executives and boards should be, too.

APPLICATION GUIDELINES FOR THE CEO

1. Use measurement not only to establish and maintain standards, but also to raise aspirations and create a new sense of what is possible.
2. The measures you track should reflect your theory of the business. Everything you measure should be either an outcome you value or something that enables an outcome you value.
3. Build measurement systems into the routine practices of your business, and teach people how to use them.

4. Educate the board and staff on public report cards and identify those with enough credibility and impact to include with your organizational standards of performance.

5. Remember the difference between meaningful and statistically significant. You want to measure and improve performance in a way that is meaningful to your organization and the people you serve.

APPLICATION GUIDELINES FOR THE BOARD

1. Look to the CEO to propose standards and measures, but do not merely rubber stamp these recommendations. Take this opportunity to clarify what behaviors and results are important to you as a board.

2. You do not want to be flooded with data. Choose measures carefully and insist that the CEO do likewise. This is an area where too much is not a good thing.

3. The most powerful measures are selected in advance and reflect your understanding of your business and your standards of performance. Occasionally, a new, meaningful measure will be developed as knowledge and understanding increases, but be wary. Post hoc measures can distract your attention from performance issues.

4. Stay alert to the information on public report cards and insist management do likewise. Do not assume the data or conclusions are accurate, but understand that others will.

5. Use internal and external scorecards as resources for performance discussions with management.

REFERENCES

Chait, R. P., W. P. Ryan, and B. E. Taylor. 2005. *Governance as Leadership: Reframing the Work of Nonprofit Boards.* Hoboken, NJ: John Wiley & Sons.

Huff, D. 1993. *How to Lie with Statistics.* New York: Norton.

Kaplan, R. S., and D. P. Norton. 2004. *Strategy Maps.* Boston: Harvard Business School Press.

————. 2001. *The Strategy-Focused Organization.* Boston: Harvard Business School Press.

————. 1996. *The Balanced Scorecard.* Boston: Harvard Business School Press.

Walton, M. 1986. *The Deming Management Method.* New York: Putnam.

CHAPTER 7

BOARD APPRAISAL
AND DEVELOPMENT

WHEN I RETURNED to consulting, one of my first engagements was to assist a hospital board that had recently completed a standardized self-evaluation. The board survey included 38 ratings on six factors: board effectiveness, strategic planning, quality and safety, medical staff relations, financial oversight, and management relations. It resulted in a statistical report more than 30 pages long. The amount of data buried the good information the report contained.

The survey employed a scale ranging from 1 ("needs significant improvement") to 5 ("outstanding"). On this survey, a 3 was "good." The board rated only three items below that level, and all three were very close to good: 2.8, 2.8, and 2.9. On the surface, it appeared the board was positive about its performance. However, I have observed a rater response bias among boards that shifts most scores up by almost a full point on a 1–5 scale where 3 is defined as "good." Therefore, any rating of 3.5 or lower would concern me, even though that is theoretically halfway between "good" and "highly effective." In this instance, discussions with the CEO and board members confirmed that there was widespread concern with items that received these ratings, even though most board members had scored performance on them as good or better.

I rank-ordered the items. Twenty-five percent were rated 3.5 or lower. Although this included items from four of the six dimensions, most items related to board effectiveness and physician relations. That's where we dug in. The board members articulated their concerns, identified targets that would represent improvements, and began specific plans to change behavior. And they stuck with it.

This is a good example of a CEO and board effectively using board self-appraisal as the starting point for improvement. They didn't stop with the appraisal. They didn't take comfort in scores that looked good. The CEO and board leaders knew issues existed, and they initiated a process that led from self-assessment to implementation of self-correction.

WHY BOARD SELF-APPRAISAL IS SO DIFFICULT

This story illustrates one reason board self-appraisal is so difficult: A response bias shows up on standardized rating forms and in discussions. Board members often hesitate to criticize their colleagues or management. This means a CEO cannot take board self-reports at face value. "Good" may not actually mean *good*; it may indicate *not so good* or *needs improvement*. "Needs improvement" could signify *this is a real problem for us.*

This does not imply that board members are attempting to deceive themselves or anyone else. Rather, they are complying with social norms that limit the clarity and directness with which people criticize one another. They are saying, "I value our relationship. I need to work with you in the future. I do not want to make anyone feel uncomfortable. I do not want to be seen as negative, and I do not want to have to justify my evaluations to others." Unless boards have practiced constructive confrontations, have confidence in the strength of their relationships, and believe candid discussion will lead to necessary and productive action, they will ordinarily not violate social conventions. CEOs and board leaders must recognize that effective evaluations start not with an evaluation form but with a shared ethic of self-improvement that outweighs the impulse to be polite.

Boards often use self-appraisal forms that exacerbate the problem. These evaluation tools can focus on aspects of the board role that fit a regulator's view of board responsibilities but do not strike the typical board member as substantive. For example, I received a form for a board I am on that asked me to comment about organizational performance on more than 90 different items. Each item referenced a valid and valuable standard of organizational performance. If any touched on the issues about which I was most concerned, however, they were overshadowed by the volume of items to be rated. Using rating scales (e.g., 1–5) or closed-ended questions (e.g., those to be answered yes or no) to identify developmental needs and opportunities is a short-cut form of self-appraisal that doesn't serve the board or the organization well, unless the evaluation is very well designed. Such forms have the merits of including everyone on the board and appearing objective. However, most healthcare and not-for-profit boards are small enough that a survey device is not needed to collect data. A CEO, board chair, or governance committee could accomplish a great deal more through direct conversation with individuals or small groups using open-ended questions. If problems of consistency, confidentiality, or comparison suggest the need for an alternative approach, consider the use of a consultant experienced in working with boards. Do not rule out questionnaires completely, but remember their limitations and do not rely solely on them.

TAKING RESPONSIBILITY FOR DEVELOPMENT

Habit 7 of Covey's *The Seven Habits of Highly Effective People* (1989) is "sharpening the saw." Although he uses it in a broader context than I do here, I specifically want to endorse his notion that this is the habit that makes the others possible. Just as individuals make themselves more effective by taking time to refresh and renew, so too can boards. Covey warns that because development is seldom an urgent issue, it often gets pushed aside by more pressing obligations. In fact, if development does become an urgent issue, it signals problems.

See Table 7.1, which is parallel to the individual board member analysis presented in Table 1.1. According to this view, development pays off whether a board begins with strong or weak board skills. In fact, I would argue that a weak board on the lower right has brighter prospects than a strong board on the upper left. Just as with individuals, a weak board with a high commitment to development can build strength, but a complacent one can grow weak quietly, escaping notice.

A CEO who wants to begin work on board development before it becomes an urgent issue needs to acquire allies on the board who share this goal. Then the CEO and chair need to organize them into a coherent force that can make an impact on the board as a whole. The best tool for this purpose is a governance committee with a charter for board development and performance improvement.

An active governance committee can dig into issues, assess performance, identify desired outcomes, and recommend improvements. With proper executive support, such a committee can key in on potential problems and improvements with greater insight and precision than most standardized self-appraisal instruments. As the members of the governance committee become skilled in their responsibilities, they set an example for the rest of the board. Through them, the board takes ownership of its development. The CEO provides consultative and administrative support but does not assume a responsibility that properly belongs to the board.

DEVELOPMENTAL PLANNING: THE SHOTGUN VERSUS THE RIFLE

A CEO's experience in planning individual development for senior executives does not translate directly to planning development

Table 7.1 Board Commitment to Development

	Low Commitment to Development	High Commitment to Development
Strong Board Skills	Complacent board; may drift into trouble	High-performing board that maximizes talent; development is important, not urgent
Weak Board Skills	Drifting and problem-prone	Troubled board in recovery mode; development is urgent and important

for the board. Effective executive development relies mainly on work assignments, secondarily on specific educational opportunities, and least on group education. However, most developmental opportunities for the board engage the board as a whole rather than individual members. (The primary exception is the grooming of board officers, described in Chapter 3.) That is the difference between the more specific targeting with a rifle and the broader scatter with a shotgun.

A shotgun approach reduces the potential impact of education but is nevertheless an important tool for CEOs and boards. Boards generally appreciate presentations by staff because they educate the board and strengthen their sense of knowledge and affiliation with the organization. Likewise, presentations by external experts or consultants (whether on-site or at conferences) help them put their own organization's issues and actions into context. Such sessions increase their self-confidence and their confidence in administration by helping them understand the present and anticipate the future more clearly. Reading materials can complement these developmental exercises, but CEOs should expect less engagement and less impact to result from reading.

In terms of potential for making a difference, board workshops and retreats score highest among shotgun approaches. In the workshop or retreat setting, the board can focus and sustain its attention better than it can under other circumstances. There is more opportunity for concentration and communication. Even the social aspects of a retreat add value since they help build trust and mutual confidence among board members. A well-run workshop or retreat produces a tangible product or plan in addition to the educational experience, so board members feel like productive contributors (which frequently does not happen in board meetings). This encourages board members to seek more opportunities to add value to the organization and the board.

CEOs should not neglect the opportunity to use individually targeted approaches, however. Perhaps the best CEO I ever witnessed in this respect was a school superintendent who made a practice of regular one-on-one interaction with his board members. I served on the board of education in his district and had breakfast with him at least once every other month. Each breakfast included discussion of an issue or two facing the school district and his perspectives on the relevant legal, regulatory, educational, political, and financial contexts. He was lobbying me, of course, but he was also educating me in a way that would not be possible in a board meeting. It gave me the opportunity to question, probe, and test alternatives without the same time constraints and other limitations that existed in the board meetings.

Most CEOs are experienced coaches. They should not overlook the opportunity to coach board members one-on-one. Other priorities may make it difficult to devote as much time to this as my superintendent did. That doesn't mean they should abandon this approach; it just means they should be more selective in terms of who they coach and on what. In contrast to the diffused and uncertain payoff of the shotgun approach, the rifle approach builds relationships, gets results, and often provides immediate feedback.

DEALING WITH DEFICIENCIES

The case study that opened this chapter provided a great example of how to solve problems effectively. The board sensed simmering discontent and hired a consultant to probe a little deeper. When the results confirmed serious issues in need of attention, they engaged another consultant skilled in board development and scheduled a special workshop focused on these concerns. They defined the problems, clarified their desired outcomes, and committed to specific steps for improvement. The CEO supported the board's self-appraisal, worked with board leaders to make the consultation as useful as possible, and organized follow-up in line with the board's priorities.

Board deficiencies generally fall into one of three categories: knowledge gaps, process problems, or commitment shortfalls. CEOs need to recognize that the "cures" for each are different. However, improving any one of these will improve the other two just as problems in one area will infect the others. For example, when knowledge and expertise grow, they reinforce commitment. When commitment is strong, the desire grows for more knowledge and skill. When board members grow frustrated by inefficient board processes, their enthusiasm wanes. And so on.

When dealing with deficiencies, consider these principles:

- Content education is easiest, and it should be a routine part of board development.
- Working on commitment is hardest because it is a by-product rather than a direct result of development activities. Pumping up commitment can have the same short-lasting impact that many so-called motivational speeches have: a short burst of enthusiasm followed by a return to the status quo.
- Dealing with process problems has the greatest potential for positive impact.

Consider a sports analogy. It can be helpful for a player to learn about the history of the sport, the great teams, and the great players. Studying the performance of winning teams and the training regimens of the outstanding players will provide strategies for success. Likewise, encouragement during practice and a fiery pre-game pep talk may energize a team to put forth maximum effort. Good coaches provide all of those things. However, a good coach must also help the players learn the fundamentals and mechanics of the sport. The coach must hone the team's performance through practice of techniques that increase individual and group speed, power, and coordination. Only then can the team perform at its maximum level and enjoy the success that follows.

APPLICATION GUIDELINES FOR THE CEO

1. Remember not to take board self-reports at face value. Just as "good" is not a good enough rating on a patient satisfaction survey, "good" signals problems, not success, on most board self-appraisals.
2. Do not overuse questionnaires as a board self-appraisal tool. Consider them a supplement to heart-to-heart conversations with committed and perceptive board members.
3. Board appraisal can be a minefield for a CEO or board chair. A governance committee has great payoffs because the board takes responsibility for itself.
4. One-on-one meetings with board members are time consuming but productive in terms of content and relationship building. Consciously decide where this fits in your list of priorities; do not let it be accidental.
5. Your board's impact will increase if you coach board members on process skills. You may need to be subtle; you do not want to be, or appear to be, self-serving. Use your allies on the governance committee.

APPLICATION GUIDELINES FOR THE BOARD

1. To improve your board and its performance, balance politeness with a determination to uncover the real issues.

2. Board self-appraisal is an area where consulting assistance can help bring important issues to the surface constructively.

3. A board committed to self-improvement has greater prospects than a stronger but more complacent board.

4. Board workshops and retreats often yield higher satisfaction and performance than routine board meetings because they allow board members to dig deeply into important issues. Encourage your board chair and CEO to make these part of your board schedule.

5. Be patient and persistent when learning new skills. Just as in sports, the method that comes naturally is not necessarily the most effective in terms of the ratio of effort to output.

REFERENCE

Covey, S. R. 1989. *The Seven Habits of Highly Effective People.* New York: Simon & Schuster.

CHAPTER 8

CEO APPRAISAL
AND DEVELOPMENT

IF THERE WAS ever a case of mixed feelings, it is the attitude of executives toward performance appraisal. They know it is important, and they insist others do it, but many drag their feet when it comes to their own appraisals. This problem is even larger for CEOs working with boards. CEOs should be role models, but their appraisals seldom stand as shining examples. Appraising the CEO is one of the board's most important responsibilities, but it is generally the CEO who must initiate the process if it is to be done well and on time.

Given their mixed feelings about appraisals, CEOs may give in to the temptation to leave well enough alone. This sets the CEO up for problems if the board's tone shifts from positive and supportive to cautious, skeptical, mistrusting, or negative. In the absence of well-done, regularly scheduled appraisals, a board evaluation of a CEO is likely to be black or white rather than a more accurate shade of gray.

LET THE SUNSHINE IN

When I was CEO, one of my board chairs was the CEO of a public institution with a board elected by the community. He was a great board chair, but his experiences with the politics of evaluation made him cautious, even minimalistic, about CEO appraisal. He knew appraisal could easily deteriorate into a political football game. Personal agendas could supplant performance as the focus, resulting in defensiveness rather than development. To prevent this, he narrowed the scope of our evaluations. He coached, questioned, and engaged with me, but didn't evaluate me except when I initiated it. I adopted his minimalist approach.

That approach wouldn't work in today's environment. It sets up boards and CEOs for trouble if their performance is called into question. CEOs serve themselves and their organizations better if their approach to their performance appraisal satisfies their needs, their boards' needs, and the needs of appropriately interested third parties.

Seventy-five to 80 percent of a CEO's appraisal should mirror the organization's objectives. Over the long haul, the CEO's successes are the organization's successes and vice versa. Whether or not this is true in a literal sense, it must be true in a practical sense. Organizations can succeed or fail in spite of their CEOs, but it is hard to assess such a situation objectively. This varies by industry and environment, of course. Some organizations have more resources at their disposal than others, and external events can skew results significantly. Nevertheless, CEOs must hold themselves accountable for overall organizational performance, and they should also expect their boards to hold them accountable.

The CEO appraisal process should start shortly after the approval of the organization's annual budget and operating plan. The CEO and the executive committee or full board should discuss how the organization's objectives and those of the CEO line up. They should

- identify where the CEO's personal involvement is most essential,
- note where qualitative assessments may take precedence over quantitative ones,

- decide how they will measure success, and
- specify how long-term goals and annual objectives will be assessed.

This is where the light should shine. Participation is critical at the starting point. Multiple perspectives are more beneficial to establishing goals and metrics than to determining whether those goals and metrics have been achieved. This also applies to the development of CEO incentive pay objectives.

CEOs and boards learn a great deal when they review what has and has not been achieved, but beginning with a shared understanding of goals and accountability enhances that learning experience. Otherwise, you can end up with the situation Bertrand Russell described when he said: "Democracy is the process by which people choose the person who'll get the blame."

BREAKING THE MOLD: BUILDING ON UNIQUE STRENGTHS

Not all CEOs are the same, despite the similar job requirements listed by many boards and search firms. I lifted these from a recent CEO posting (and didn't even include all of the expected priorities and qualities):

> quality care is the number one priority; innovation or early adoption of new technology; continuous improvement in employee and physician satisfaction; challenging existing paradigms; proven record of executing strategies, goals, and tactics; visionary leadership and an ability to successfully operationalize; collaborative strategic direction process; ability to effectively communicate the strategic vision and imperatives; financial acumen with proven strong analytical and technical abilities; decisive in financial decision making; business acumen; proven understanding of the functional disciplines; collaborative relationships with physicians; trust and support for every employee; understanding and supporting the

greater good of the community; meeting community healthcare needs beyond the hospital; ability to support the Board and Board leadership; success earning and deserving a Board's trust.

There is a sameness to the stated expectations across multiple organizations because of the natural desire for the CEO to be able to do it all, to meet everyone's expectations, even if they are contradictory. Every recruiter and board starts with the professed desire to match the individual to the specific internal and external challenges of the organization, but they often end up with a grab bag of individual perspectives that rarely add up to a solid job description.

This can be a problem when it comes time to appraise CEOs. Individuals cannot balance and excel in all of these expectations. In fact, attempting to do so is a prescription for underperformance. Job descriptions for CEOs list multiple tasks that must be accomplished with a reasonable degree of proficiency. This leads to minimal standards of performance or expectations. However, at some point the CEO will need to develop strategies and operational plans for the organization. These goals and objectives are likely to demand more than a minimal level of performance, and are where the appraisal of CEOs should focus.

CEOs should hold themselves accountable for the nuts and bolts of the work, and their boards should do likewise. However, they commit a serious error if appraisal begins and ends there. They fall prey to mediocrity if they spend too much time rectifying flaws that are not critical. Savvy CEOs and boards will identify the CEO's outstanding talents and match them to specific opportunities or challenges the organization faces. CEOs and boards need to share their aspirations and align their efforts to achieve something special, rather than just checking off boxes on a list of standard expectations and generically desirable traits.

In *Now, Discover Your Strengths*, Buckingham and Clifton (2001, 7) report that most organizations were built on flawed assumptions about people, including that "each person's greatest room for growth is in his or her areas of greatest weakness." They contrast this with the finding that great managers followed a markedly different assumption, namely that "each person's greatest room for growth is in the areas of his or her greatest strength" (Buckingham and Clifton 2001, 8). Therefore, they recommend you start with these questions when considering your own development: "What are your strengths? How can you capitalize on them? What are your most powerful combinations? Where do they take you?" (Buckingham and Clifton 2001, 10). Appraisals and development that begin there set the stage for great accomplishments.

DECIDING WHAT NOT TO DO

After a long list of leadership competencies, the CEO job specs quoted earlier ended with this performance expectation: "Proven ability to focus, align, and integrate organizational priorities." Focus is one of the qualifications missing in the list itself, and that omission reflects the state of affairs challenging most CEOs today. Managers have always contended with a multitude of demands. Mintzberg (1973) observed in *The Nature of Managerial Work* that senior managers felt stressed by the multiple, open-ended, and unending demands of work. Many fell into an "activity-trap." They raced from activity to activity and controlled little of what they did—and that was before the Internet, e-mail, cell phones, and BlackBerries demanded 24/7 accessibility and responsiveness.

As Peter Drucker (1985) writes in *The Effective Executive*, "There are always more important contributions to be made than there is time available to make them . . . (108). The job is, however, not to set priorities. That is easy. Everybody can do it. The reason why so few executives concentrate is the difficulty of setting 'posteriorities'—that is, deciding what tasks not to tackle—and of sticking to the decision . . . (109–110). It is much easier to draw up a nice list of top priorities and then to hedge by trying to do 'just a little bit' of everything else as well. This makes everybody happy. The only drawback is, of course, that nothing whatever gets done" (111).

When I first became a CEO, I had the good fortune of working with an enlightened executive committee. When I sat down with them to discuss my objectives, I had reduced the multiple-page list of performance standards to five categories of bulleted goals that filled a page and a half. They looked at it and asked, "Which three or four things are most essential and will make the greatest impact on the organization this year?" I had made a good start in the right direction, but they impelled me to focus even more. More important, they made me commit to the essential few. Like any CEO, I had to keep a lot of balls in the air as I juggled competing priorities, but I didn't have to keep them *all* in the air. What's more, I shared an understanding of priorities—and posteriorities—with the executive committee.

CEOs and their boards need to decide when "good enough" is indeed good enough. Without a shared understanding of priorities and measures of success, CEO appraisal and development will swing from hot topic to hot topic, from yesterday's urgent issue to today's. CEOs need to focus on the vital few. They cannot be all things for all people, not even all board members. This is both a practical and a philosophical position. As Voltaire said, "The perfect is the enemy of the good."

"MAYBE IT WILL GO AWAY"

Each time I visit my dentist for a checkup and lie back in his chair, I read a little decal affixed to his dental lamp right where his patients will see it. It says: "The five most dangerous words— *Maybe it will go away.*" It is a lesson CEOs and boards should remember when they discover they have conflicting expectations for the CEO's performance.

Boards and CEOs can find themselves in conflict regarding focus, philosophy, and outcomes. Board members may also disagree among themselves. Ignoring such conflicts, hoping they will just go away, only creates problems down the road. It is like the mechanic said in the old Fram oil filter commercial: "You can pay me now [for a new filter], or you can pay me later [when your car breaks down]."

Consultants bring hidden agendas and unspoken objectives into the light of day. They do the same with unreconciled conflicts. CEOs should learn from their example. It is always to CEOs' advantage to clarify expectations, especially where they note conflicts, whether overt or lying beneath the surface. If they perceive that sensitivities are great or the risks are too high, they may choose to rely on the assistance of an external consultant—especially if the conflicting expectations are wearing away at the mutual trust and confidence of the board and CEO. Under ordinary circumstances, however, CEOs, acting as consultants to their own boards, can model adult behavior by respectfully raising such issues for mutual consideration and candid dialogue.

APPLICATION GUIDELINES FOR THE CEO

1. Be a role model for performance appraisal. Recognize that it is in the organization's interest and your own best interest to not let this practice be absent or perfunctory.

2. Coordinate the planning of your performance appraisal with the annual planning process for the organization. It provides one more opportunity to reach agreement with board leadership about the key drivers of organizational performance and their expectations for your leadership.

3. Review the questions suggested by Buckingham and Clifton (2001). These are the keys to building on your strengths to achieve organizational success.

4. Beware of the activity trap. There will be many explicit demands and implicit expectations for you to do it all. If you let this happen, your overall achievements will decrease while your stress and energy expenditure increase.

5. Remember the five most dangerous words: "Maybe it will go away." Use external assistance if you need to, but do not let yourself be skewered later by conflicting expectations that need to be addressed now.

APPLICATION GUIDELINES FOR THE BOARD

1. Your organization should have a policy for CEO appraisal, and it should be followed. Although you may depend on the CEO to set the agenda for the board, treat this as seriously as the annual audit. It should not be a discretionary activity.

2. Hold your CEO accountable for organizational performance. Being supportive and holding an executive accountable are not mutually exclusive. Refer to Chapter 6 for more advice regarding measurement.

3. If you as the board cannot reconcile your own differences and priorities, you set your CEO up for mediocrity and, perhaps, outright failure. Work with your CEO to ensure a shared sense of the key success factors for the organization and the level of performance expected on each.

4. Know what your "posteriorities" are—those goals that are worthwhile in the abstract but can be sacrificed to ensure excellent performance on priorities.

5. If you and your CEO find yourselves in unresolved conflicts about expectations, get help. If you do not deal with conflict constructively, it will erode your mutual trust and confidence, and you may end up hiring a search consultant instead.

REFERENCES

Buckingham, M., and D. O. Clifton. 2001. *Now, Discover Your Strengths.* New York: Free Press.

Drucker, P. F. 1985. *The Effective Executive.* New York: Harper Colophon.

Mintzberg, H. 1973. *The Nature of Managerial Work.* New York: HarperCollins.

CHAPTER 9

MANAGING PROBLEMS AND CRISES

LIKE EXECUTIVE WORK, most board work falls into one of three categories: improving the organization, maintaining operations, or managing problems. And as is true for an executive, a board consistently mired in firefighting is a board in an unsustainable, dysfunctional situation. However, no executive or board is ever likely to find itself problem-free. CEOs and boards can reduce the frequency of occurrence, they can limit the size and scope of problems and mitigate the effects, but they cannot escape the inescapable. Problems come with the territory. Common problems include deviations from plan, conflicts or potential conflicts of interest, systemic problems highlighted by complaints or audits, and crises—both real and of the public relations variety.

DEVIATIONS FROM THE PLAN

In 2007, 11 major league baseball players batted .330 or better. The top batter, Magglio Ordonez of the Detroit Tigers, hit .363, or a bit better than one hit every three times at bat. Ten other players had perfect averages of 1.000, but those ten had a total of 13 at bats all season—not enough to qualify any of them for consideration as a hit leader. In baseball, as in life, if you want to be perfect, you have to attempt almost nothing and quit while you're ahead.

I do not think a batting average is calculable for CEOs and boards, but if it were, I am confident no one would approach 1.000. CEOs need to make constant adjustments as the environment changes and as they learn the effects of their actions and the outcomes of their plans. Enlightened managers do not expect perfection. Instead, they build systems to anticipate, prevent, or minimize problems; detect deviations from plan; understand what those deviations mean; and implement corrective actions. They use deviations from plan as a key learning tool. They improve their aim by analyzing their misses.

Although mistakes present great opportunities and motivation for learning, no one likes to make them. It is possible to intellectually embrace mistakes while rejecting them emotionally. Unfortunately, the first response to a mistake is more often "Whose fault is it?" than "What can we learn from this?" CEOs working as consultants to their boards (and as leaders of their management teams) need to change this approach. See Hofmann and Perry (2005), *Management Mistakes in Healthcare*, for an in-depth review and helpful suggestions.

In a complex environment such as modern healthcare, balanced scorecards or strategy maps as recommended by Kaplan and Norton (1996) are essential management tools. As noted in Chapter 6, they advise organizations to link measurements to their theory of the business. For example, what measurable operational improvements lead to what customer outcomes, producing what financial results? Deviations from plan at any of these levels provide diagnostic feedback to leaders and point the way to corrective actions.

CEOs should ensure a shared understanding of and agreement on the key measures of success. They need to help the board recognize how the measures link together and how management will use feedback to adjust tactics and reallocate resources. Boards, for their part, need to let their CEOs know which goals and measures are highest priority for them.

In one hospital, for example, medication errors exceeded target for several quarters running. The CEO and board agreed that this level of performance was unsatisfactory. Their first efforts at correction did not pay off, and the lack of progress made everyone uncomfortable, from board, through CEO and management, to medical and nursing staff leadership. However, the CEO did not let this discourage him. He continued to measure, report deviations to the board, and institute still more corrective actions. The measurement, corrective action plans, resource allocations, and follow-up remained a standing item on the board agenda until together they achieved success and confirmed that it was lasting. In this instance, combined CEO and board attention ensured the problem remained a priority until it was resolved.

CONFLICTS OF INTEREST

Conflicts of interest put a different kind of stress on the CEO and board. Anyone can deal with conflicts of interest that involve people with no ongoing relationship. But conflicts of interest are unpleasant challenges when they involve people who respect each other and must continue to work together—such as boards.

Nevertheless, boards are the primary managers of potential conflicts of interest within their ranks. This is an inherent responsibility of self-governance. They cannot wash their hands of it or delegate it fully to administration. However, as in most other situations involving boards, CEOs can take an active role in setting the stage and supporting implementation.

A board's work would be easier if it were able to draw a bright line separating permissible and impermissible relationships. Unfortunately, despite the well-meaning advice of "zero tolerance" advocates, such an approach is unrealistic. Hospitals and health systems are often among the largest enterprises in their communities. Their business and professional transactions encompass a broad segment of the community, especially among those with the skills and background to serve on healthcare boards. Since boards cannot eliminate potential conflicts by fiat, they must manage them with rules and culture. The fact that a bright line cannot be drawn does not mean no line can be drawn.

The first step is to acknowledge that conflicts are expected, so they can be named, defined, and described in board policies. Boards that accept the inevitability of conflicts of interest can deal with them in a nondisruptive, nonprejudicial, business-like fashion. When boards treat conflicts as an aberration, calling attention to a potential conflict feels like an attack or a statement of distrust. On the New York State Hospital Review and Planning Council, provider members routinely submit their conflicts to the chair before each meeting. As each agenda item comes up, the chair announces the members with an interest and the members with a conflict. The former can participate in discussion, but not vote; the latter leave the room for the entire discussion and the vote. This system does not resolve all issues, but it deals with the bulk of potential conflicts smoothly and publicly and with no ill will.

To avoid the extremes of head-in-the-sand neglect and zero tolerance, CEOs and boards should create policies and practices to bring potential conflicts to the awareness of all members and handle them procedurally rather than personally. By working proactively, they minimize the likelihood of conflict-of-interest problems undermining credibility or rising to crisis level. Because conflict of interest is subject to legal and regulatory scrutiny, CEOs and boards should seek legal counsel as they develop their policies and procedures.

WHERE THERE'S SMOKE, THERE'S FIRE

Few things move a board from governance to management more quickly than complaints, negative reviews, or audit findings. Even board members committed to keeping their hands out of management find their resolve tested when they receive complaints or concerns from legitimate sources.

Complaints from individuals, even if they are incidental and anecdotal, can make an impact out of proportion to their actual numbers. Board members, like most people, are affected more strongly by flesh-and-blood stories than by pages of statistics. Reports of shortcomings can trigger powerful urges to intervene. Board members who are already skeptical about management's performance may quickly generalize specific situations to draw conclusions about overall performance.

Negative reviews by accrediting agencies, auditors, or other outsiders may have less impact than individual complaints. Board members will often side with their own institution against an outside organization. Patterns of problems or shortcomings, however, will change that. CEOs can find themselves on the defensive as board members demand corrective action. With repetition, the likelihood grows that board members will propose or direct specific actions rather than continue to delegate that responsibility to management.

Despite management protests to the contrary, the board is not wrong to investigate negative feedback carefully. Organizations usually have an institutional bias toward maintaining the status quo. Most will dismiss the legitimacy of complaints unless the organizational culture is positive about learning from mistakes. Problems can fester longer than necessary without a system to track issues and monitor resolution. Boards serve the organization poorly if they use each negative situation as a signal to become personally involved, but they also serve poorly if they allow inertia to rule. Newton's first law of motion is as applicable to organizations as it is to objects: a body at rest tends to remain at rest and a body in motion tends to remain in motion—unless an external force acts on it. CEOs serve their boards, their organizations, and themselves well if they help the board understand and use problems constructively.

REAL AND/OR PR CRISES

Crises happen in healthcare. Some are real (such as malfunctioning equipment leading to patient injury or death). Others result from perceptions (such as a false allegation of misconduct causing a rash of negative publicity). In either case, the board, as the body ultimately responsible for hospital quality, and the CEO, as the chief executive, must resolve the situation. A crisis will quickly demonstrate how much mutual trust and respect the CEO and board have.

As a hospital VP, I witnessed such a situation firsthand. An allegation of misconduct made to a regulator who harbored an old grudge against our hospital led to a massive review of patient cases. The resulting report distorted the facts, but that problem was magnified by the hospital's poor or incomplete documentation. The pattern of evidence seemed to point to outrageous levels of negligence. The results leaked, and our external support vanished. However, our board stood by us, which was a testament not only to their character but also to the open and mutually respectful relationships the CEO had created.

In a crisis, communication to the board and leadership by the board, both of which follow a classic S pattern as shown in Figure 9.1, are essential. Communication with the board must happen as soon as the problem passes a minimum threshold of importance. The need for communication increases as the seriousness of the problem increases. Active involvement by the board should grow parallel to the communication, but at a lower level unless the issue is very serious. When the issue involves the core mission, activities, or reputation of the organization, the board as representatives of the community—the ultimate owners of the organization—must take the lead in ensuring resolution and assuring the community that the situation will be corrected.

CEOs following the consultant model will communicate with the board to ensure trust and mutual understanding and to build the board's knowledge base and confidence. Without two-way communication, a board may either intervene when

Figure 9.1 Communication and Leadership Should Increase Rapidly as Seriousness Increases

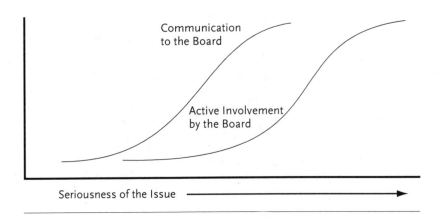

it's inappropriate or fail to take leadership when its active involvement is needed.

Good systems and careful planning will eliminate some problems, but not all. CEOs and boards should remember these ABCs:

- Anticipate that problems will occur.
- Build systems and relationships in advance to ensure problems are raised and managed, not minimized or ignored.
- Communicate early and often.

APPLICATION GUIDELINES FOR THE CEO

1. Do not become mired in firefighting, but expect problems and build systems to unearth them, correct them, and track the results.
2. If you construct your balanced scorecard so it reflects your theory of the business, deviations from target will help you adjust tactics and refine implementation.

3. Help the board develop systems and processes for identifying and managing conflicts of interest. It is their responsibility, but you are their consultant.

4. Humans and their organizations seek comfortable equilibrium, so problems are often fixed only temporarily, until people revert back to their old habits. If you do not build tracking mechanisms to ensure lasting change, you will find yourself dealing with the same problems again and again and losing credibility with your board.

5. Keep your board informed about significant problems, but do not request their action until you need it. Help them learn the difference between a report and a request.

APPLICATION GUIDELINES FOR THE BOARD

1. Make sure you speak up early about the results most important to you as a board. This will help with selecting the right measures, and you will know when organizational efforts hit or miss.

2. Preventing conflicts of interest and dealing with them when they occur are your responsibility, not management's. Be serious and proactive about this.

3. Be careful about jumping to conclusions concerning a complaint. You should not be blindly loyal to management, but unless they have proven unreliable, you should always start by giving them the benefit of the doubt.

4. Require management to follow up on problems and to ensure corrective action is lasting. Set this expectation explicitly when audits or external reviews result in citations or recommendations. Create your own mechanisms to track adherence to this direction.

5. Be prepared to take the heat publicly in the event of a serious crisis, but also be prepared to make some heat privately within the organization to protect the interests of the public.

REFERENCES

Hofmann, P. B., and F. Perry. 2005. *Management Mistakes in Healthcare: Identification, Correction and Prevention.* Cambridge, UK: Cambridge University Press.

Kaplan, R. S., and D. P. Norton. 1996. *The Balanced Scorecard.* Boston: Harvard Business School Press.

SECTION III

HOW?

CHAPTER 10

BUILDING RELATIONSHIPS

E. E. CUMMINGS (1968) wrote "one's not half two. It's two are halves of one." It makes no sense mathematically, but it is a truth of relationships. Two people in a relationship form a new unit that is different from the addition of one and one.

Years ago, I reviewed the work of a number of total quality management teams. When I compared the teams, I learned something that seemed counterintuitive. The teams who had plunged immediately into their work were less successful than those who had spent time getting to know each other as individuals and building a sense of themselves together as a team. The less successful teams were completely task-focused. The more successful teams had also attended to relationships. This may not seem like an earth-shaking insight, but consider how it violates our notions of the primacy of work effort.

ADAM KAHANE'S INSIGHT

Years later, I slipped back into my old way of thinking without realizing it. As a CEO, I had to solve tough problems, and I was eager to learn new approaches. I heard about a book by Adam

Kahane (2004) called *Solving Tough Problems.* I figured it would be just what I needed. It was, but it wasn't what I expected.

Adam Kahane solved *tough* problems, problems that dwarfed my own as CEO. He was the facilitator who worked with representatives of the African National Congress and the South African government to help plan for a post-apartheid South Africa. The core of his work was a scenario-planning approach. However, he did some things that initially baffled me and revealed my impulse to put tasks before relationships.

One morning, during a day-and-a-half work session Kahane was facilitating for the two opposing parties, they suspended their formal activities to watch a World Cup game in which the South African team was playing. I was aghast. *What? They stopped working on their mission to end apartheid to watch football?*

That morning marked a breakthrough. They returned to their work with a sense of having something in common. They had begun to build a bridge across their differences of history, race, power, and economics. They moved ahead with greater willingness to see from each other's perspectives. Kahane went on to work in other tough situations and observed similar breakthroughs. As soon as people made personal connections beyond their formal organizational roles, they discovered more innovative and more effective ways to get things done. Relationships provided a foundation for leaping ahead.

TRUST, CONFIDENCE, AND RESPECT

Jeffrey Sonnenfeld (2002) captured the same idea in the title of his article "What Makes Great Boards Great: It's Not Rules and Regulations. It's the Way People Work Together." He examined the usual prescriptions and concluded, "So if following good-governance regulatory recipes doesn't produce good boards, what does? The key isn't structural, it's social. . . . Team members develop mutual respect; because they respect one another, they develop trust; because they trust one another, they share difficult information. . . ." (Sonnenfeld 2002, 109).

Picture a suspension bridge. Each cable is made up of smaller cables, each similarly constructed from still smaller cables. Wound together, they have the capacity to support not only the bridge but all the traffic crossing over it. The cables are strong, yet they have the flexibility they need to function under changing circumstances. When board members develop relationships of mutual trust and respect, it is like weaving the cables of a bridge.

The time to build trust and respect is *before* it is needed. A CEO should develop strength in the board during periods of progress. Then, when the inevitable problems arise, the board members will already have the mutual regard that will enable them to work together. The board members must be ready and willing to stand by the organization and each other, and not scatter when the first pressures hit them.

Progress is evident when board members ask each other questions with respect and when they are willing to disagree with each other and accommodate each other, as circumstances require. Because they recognize a common commitment and purpose, but even more because they feel a personal link, they are willing to give the benefit of the doubt when they disagree. They are willing to listen to alternative points of view rather than automatically classify someone who disagrees with them as ignorant or misguided.

PERSONAL REGARD—MEMBER TO MEMBER

As CEO, how do you create a sense of trust among board members? How do you build mutual respect? How do you engender a spirit of personal regard? These questions bring us back to Adam Kahane's insight. You attend not only to task issues but also to relationships.

Table 10.1 Intrinsic, Extrinsic, and Hybrid Approaches to Building Trust and Personal Regard Among Board Members

Approach	Example/Why
Intrinsic (work)	Intrinsic approaches build relationships by providing recognition of the contributions and initiatives of others and by creating work settings where people will get to know each other's strengths.
• Appreciation	"Ann, I appreciate your thinking on this; it has helped us make progress more quickly than we could have otherwise."
• Building on ideas	"Bill, I like your idea. What would you think if we extended it by combining it with Carl's suggestion?"
• Inquiry	"Diane, I am not sure I understand your comment. Please tell me more about the reasoning that prompted it."
• Respectful disagreement	"Ed, I think your idea would move us forward quickly, but I am concerned that it would conflict with our other goals in this area. How do you think we could reconcile these priorities?"
• Task force and committee assignments	In addition to recognizing interests, competencies, and developmental needs, assignments can be made so that specific members get experience in working closely with each other.
Extrinsic (play)	Extrinsic approaches build relationships by providing opportunities for members to learn about each other personally apart from their board roles and tasks. These connections can be very effective in building goodwill.

See Table 10.1 for a dozen methods to increase interpersonal understanding, respect, and regard. I call these intrinsic, extrinsic, and hybrid approaches, or more simply, work, play, and both approaches.

A CEO who builds or enhances personal relationships among board members will be rewarded by the board's strength in times of crisis. However, before the task is completed, the board may

Table 10.1 *Continued*

Approach	Example/ Why
• Activities	Inviting board members to attend or participate in sporting events or community activities can provide fun, engaging, and neutral opportunities to share likes and interests.
• Meals	Group meals provide opportunities for informal discussion. Etiquette and traditions around meals support harmony and friendship.
• Parties and celebrations	A convivial atmosphere can extend beyond the time frame of the party and become a positive shared experience.
• Social hour	Time set aside for rest and refreshment lets people shift their focus from tasks to relationships. This also helps sustain energy.
Hybrid (both)	Some work activities can build knowledge and skills while creating occasions for positive social interaction.
• Conferences	Conferences provide an intense learning experience and frequently include several of the extrinsic approaches listed above.
• Retreats	A well-designed board retreat can accomplish more relationship building and task accomplishment in a day than might occur in months of typical board meetings.
• Travel	Travel for learning or benchmarking purposes creates opportunities for social interaction in addition to the formal task objectives because of the "non-productive" time that travel normally entails.

find itself in an unproductive situation where members value harmony over effectiveness and avoid conflicts for fear of harming fragile interpersonal relationships. The goal is to develop enough mutual respect that board members view disagreements as constructive and enough mutual confidence that they can challenge each other's ideas without ego or ill will.

PERSONAL REGARD—
BETWEEN MEMBERS AND STAFF

Because the CEO is the only direct employee of the board, some CEOs and boards believe no other employee should have a relationship with the board or that the CEO should moderate relationships between the board and other employees. If they act on those beliefs, they limit the potential energy and impact of the board and the organization.

Admittedly, direct relationships between board members and staff have their risks. Some staff members may take advantage of their board contacts to advocate for positions, proposals, or programs outside the proper management and board processes. They may deliberately circumvent the CEO to push their agendas. When a CEO is left out of the loop, organizational efficiency and effectiveness can suffer. The staff members can gain short-term victories, but at the cost of strained relationships with their peers and the CEO. Likewise, board members who feel they have an inside source may improperly second-guess the CEO and subvert the board process. Such board members are more likely to cross the line between governance and management. Ironically, board members and staff members who behave this way may feel particularly self-righteous and believe their actions are in the best interest of the organization. However, they are individually taking on roles that rightfully belong to the board and CEO, often operating on hidden agendas rather than public ones.

Given those risks, why should a CEO promote relationships between board members and staff? Strong mutual regard and trust help the organization pursue an active, assertive agenda in troubled times. When board members have confidence in the staff and the CEO, they have a fuller context for establishing priorities and making difficult decisions. When staff have confidence in the board, they can better understand and accept the board's role in direction setting and decision making. Staff members and board members are less apt to attribute negative motivations or apply negative evaluations to others they regard positively.

CEOs set the stage for positive relationships with the way they speak about the members of the board in the staff's presence, and vice versa. CEOs who want their staff to be recognized provide opportunities for them to present to the board and explicitly share appreciation for their accomplishments. Smart CEOs share credit liberally and specifically. They also assign key staff as support to board committees and task forces to create opportunities for them to work together. They use the intrinsic and extrinsic approaches listed above. The goal is to align the talents and energies of the board and staff by supplementing work roles with relationship-based trust and respect.

APPLICATION GUIDELINES FOR THE CEO

1. Recognize your responsibility for facilitating relationships. You do not need to act as an activities director, but if you want a strong, productive team, do not neglect this dimension.

2. Make a point of identifying and sharing connections between people to help them build relationships.

3. Model the behaviors you want to see, especially the intrinsic approaches described earlier.

4. Be alert to the danger of conflict avoidance as board members develop positive relationships. Help them use their positive regard to disagree respectfully.

5. As you help build constructive relationships between staff and board, specifically explain to staff what you are doing and your rationale. This will keep them from misunderstanding the continuing differences in roles and responsibilities among staff, CEO, and board.

APPLICATION GUIDELINES FOR THE BOARD

1. Do not be afraid to have fun. Some boards want to maintain an appearance of hard, conscientious work. As a result, they actively avoid the extrinsic and hybrid approaches that do so much to advance board effectiveness.

2. Take an active role in building relationships with your fellow board members; do not leave it up to the CEO or board chair alone.

3. When you disagree with fellow board members, remember to give them the benefit of the doubt. This signals respect for their experiences and ideas.

4. Practice the intrinsic approaches in board discussions. You will hear better and learn more, and other members will value your contributions more.

5. Learn about staff members and enjoy your contacts with them, but be alert to—and resist—the temptations that may lead you or them to step across important organizational boundaries.

REFERENCES

Cummings, E. E. 1968. *Poems 1923–1954*. New York: Harcourt, Brace & World.

Kahane, A. 2004. *Solving Tough Problems*. San Francisco: Berrett-Koehler.

Sonnenfeld, J. 2002. "What Makes Great Boards Great." *Harvard Business Review* 80 (September): 106–113.

CHAPTER 11

BOARD MEETINGS

WHY DO WE have board meetings? Few people ask because board meetings are just a fact of organizational life. However, this question is ready-made for the 5 Whys. The 5 Whys is a problem-solving tool used in Total Quality Management and Six Sigma to identify the root cause of a problem. I also use it to quickly work through layers of ideas. Asking "why?" repeatedly can uncover the assumptions or reasons behind a policy or practice.

For example: *Why do we have board meetings?* So the board can work together as a group. *Why as a group?* Because working together is more effective than working separately. *Why is it more effective?* Because board members can share perspectives and respond to each other's ideas. *Why is that important?* Because you should consider important issues from multiple perspectives. *Why?* Because different perspectives help you develop a fuller, more accurate understanding of complex issues and make decisions more people can accept. And so on, if necessary.

Obviously, not everyone would ask and answer the questions the same way. The 5 Whys can lead you down multiple roads, including dead ends, depending on how the questions are phrased and answered. The 5 Whys is a thinking aid, not a scientific method. Nevertheless, it helps you go beneath the surface and reveals a train of thought. In the example above, it makes my own cause-and-effect reasoning explicit.

Based on my experience, I believe boards make better, wiser decisions when they share perspectives, and face-to-face meetings are the best way to accomplish this. Helping such meetings work effectively, capturing the full potential of boards, is a challenge for CEOs. Just because groups *can* be more effective than individuals does not necessarily mean they *will* be. All of the chapters in Section III ("How?") are devoted to this challenge.

PARTICIPATION: HOW MUCH IS ENOUGH? HOW MUCH IS TOO MUCH?

In a January 2007 article in *Trustee* magazine, "Making the Case for Conflict," I wrote: "If CEOs sincerely want the full benefit of their boards, they should regard unanimity as a sign of trouble, not progress. . . . If trustees are always in complete agreement with the CEO and with one another, then where is the added value of having a board? . . . Particularly in a rapidly changing environment, board and management teams that have multiple talents and perspectives have much greater adaptive capabilities than do homogeneous teams" (McGinn 2007a, 32).

However, the desire to avoid conflict or time-draining discussions can lead otherwise independent people to censor themselves and discourage dissent. When this happens on a board, the board loses its most important resource and its reason for being: the breadth of experiences, insights, and perspectives of a diverse group of talented individuals.

I like to use the image of a teeter-totter as a guide for individual participation in groups. When two people on a teeter-totter are in harmony, they rise and fall in rhythm. They may have to adjust their position or energy output to keep the teeter-totter in motion, but when they find balance, they can lift their bodies with little effort and return to the ground gently and safely. To keep it going, however, they must maintain this balance.

Each member of a group, not just the leaders, is responsible for the group's success. Members contribute to the balance and effective performance of the group by neither dominating nor withdrawing from discussion and interaction. Through active participation, they ensure the group has access to their talents. Through moderation, they ensure others' talents have the opportunity to shine.

Although each member shares responsibility, the chair and CEO need to establish a climate for constructive engagement and model such behaviors themselves. One CEO I know often frames a discussion topic by providing diametrically opposite views on the issue. He reports that this encourages board members to express their own varied opinions and rationales. Approaches like this lead to better discussions and stronger, more informed support for decisions with less passive compliance and second-guessing.

BOARD AGENDA CALENDAR

Bazerman and Watkins (2004) wrote an insightful book with the apt title *Predictable Surprises*. We are often surprised by things we would have seen coming if we were not so busy maintaining the status quo and avoiding temporary discomfort. Bazerman and Watkins focused on major negative events or disasters, but board meetings can also include predictable surprises. I have frequently seen two types of items on board agendas: (1) routine items the CEO includes in every meeting without questioning their purpose and (2) whatever topic happens to be hot at the time. In the latter instance, CEOs and boards react to the time pressure to make decisions as if the demands of the annual planning and budgeting cycle or external reviews, for example, were a surprise to them.

A productive alternative I have seen less frequently involves planning an annual board agenda calendar. If the board and the CEO identify the topics the board will discuss and create a plan to review them in a sensible sequence and aligned with decision points over the course of a year, the board's work has the potential for greater impact. With a calendar in place, committee chairs can anticipate when they must deal with time-sensitive items for which their committees are responsible. They can work with management to organize committee schedules to ensure timely and complete reviews in advance of a topic appearing on the full board agenda.

Additionally, if the CEO and the board plan discussions with an annual perspective in mind, they will likely find there is in fact not enough time to cover all of the topics they want to include. This creates an opportunity to make conscious choices about organizational and board needs and priorities. Many prefer, however, to avoid these decisions by planning each meeting as it occurs. This is simpler and less demanding, but it fosters a reactive approach to decision making, decreases the likelihood of timely and thorough preparation, and engenders vague dissatisfaction about lack of progress. That's another predictable surprise.

IDD: INFORMATION, DISCUSSION, AND DECISION

"Just what do you think you are doing?" my mother used to ask me. It is not a bad question to ask CEOs and boards during their meetings. Are you providing information, discussing an issue, or making a decision? Each of these has its place in meetings, but the three need to be kept in balance. Moreover, it is essential that members know which one they are doing at a given point in the meeting.

Information

Providing information is usually a one-way street. Often the CEO or a senior staff member updates the board on current happenings, products or services, or emerging technologies. Usually the appropriate role for the board is to listen and ask questions. In some cases, however, board members have specific expertise and knowledge they can share. Information sharing is an important part of a board meeting. Problems occur when the one-way transmission occupies so much time that discussions get shortchanged or decisions get rushed or deferred. Moreover, too much information sharing can create passivity on the board's part. Frustration and resentment can boil over if the members feel information sharing takes time away from governance work. This gives information sharing an undeservedly bad reputation.

Discussion

If the teeter-totter model is working well, a board discussion can be effective and energizing. When board members have the opportunity to approach an issue from multiple angles, share their perspectives and ideas, and listen carefully to each other, they can develop fresh, new insights into difficult problems or challenges. There are three stages to many such discussions:

1. An initial, brainstorming stage where board members toss out multiple ideas
2. An intermediate, groping stage where board members try to cope with the disparity of opinions
3. A concluding, convergent stage where board members begin to find the themes that tie their ideas together

The first and third stages are fun, but the middle stage is sometimes called the "groan zone" because it can be frustrating and difficult. A CEO can advise the board on group process to help them better understand the dynamics of discussion. This will lessen their frustration or impatience and help them achieve a satisfying resolution, if not actual closure.

Decision

Ultimately, a board makes decisions. CEOs should make sure their boards understand which discussions must lead to decisions. Normally, CEOs signal these as action items on the agenda and accompany supporting materials with a management recommendation. Without such clarity, however, board members may misinterpret the intention as information or discussion only. Watch the dynamics in a board meeting. If impatience or frustration is rising, or if people are working at cross-purposes, check the agenda. Is it clear to participants whether the board is to be receiving information, engaging in discussion, or reaching a decision? Making this clear is the CEO's and chair's responsibility, but any board member can raise the issue if the agenda leaves any doubt.

BOARD RETREATS

Because of the amount of time set aside for them, board retreats provide opportunities to dive more deeply into issues. The right setting removes distractions and allows participants greater concentration. A retreat can help participants escape from routine patterns of thinking and approach problems freshly by providing an alternative to the usual meeting format. If a board has gotten into a rut, a retreat is a way out.

A good retreat also creates a climate for improved communication by using a different meeting venue and adjusting the pace and rhythm of the agenda. It is harder, for example, to keep talking in generalities for a full day than for a couple of hours. Moreover, mealtimes and other scheduled social activities add personal communication to business communication. These interactions build the trust and confidence among trustees (discussed in Chapter 10) that improves board effectiveness.

In not-for-profit healthcare, CEOs may hesitate to add yet another activity to the schedules of their already busy and dedicated board members. Board members may face the prospect of an additional day or more away from work or family with reluctance or even resistance. A CEO should respect board members' other commitments. However, a CEO who fails to use the opportunities presented by a good retreat shortchanges the organization and the board members. A retreat enables board members to step out of the action–reaction cycle and put threats and opportunities into context. Most board members find a good retreat so productive that their energy and enthusiasm grow rather than wane as the retreat progresses. Some boards include one or more retreats on the calendar each year.

In the May 2007 issue of *Trustee* magazine, I described the factors that make retreats so valuable: enabling concentration, improving communication, making connections between ideas, gaining perspective, and producing organized output (McGinn 2007b). A poorly conceived or run retreat, like a poorly conceived or run board meeting, is a waste of time. A good retreat, however, has tangible payoffs. In return for the investment, board members can identify paths for organizational progress while building stronger bonds with their colleagues, both of which they find rewarding.

APPLICATION GUIDELINES FOR THE CEO

1. Do not accept board meetings as a routine. Plan agendas that maximize the benefit of your board members' knowledge and experiences. If the board gets into a rut, change the format and topics to get them out.

2. Apply the teeter-totter model to yourself. It is easy for CEOs to dominate meetings. Model the participation style you'd like to see in other participants. See also Chapter 4.

3. Create an annual calendar for board agendas to ensure organizational priorities receive sufficient attention. Arrange them in a sequence that supports good, timely discussions and decision making. Always leave room, however, for unanticipated items.

4. When you identify agenda items as information, discussion, or decision, watch for two problems: an overrepresentation of information items and information items disguised as discussion items. Information is necessary, but discussion and decision are at the heart of what a board should do.

5. Invest in board retreats. Commit to them at least annually. Consider the lessons of Chapter 10 as you structure board retreats.

APPLICATION GUIDELINES FOR THE BOARD

1. Know what you expect from board meetings. Do not passively accept the process because that is the way it has always been done.

2. Check yourself on the teeter-totter model in board meetings. If you are not engaging, you are depriving your colleagues and the organization of the benefit of your knowledge and experiences. If you are dominating, you are depriving yourself and the organization of the benefit of others' knowledge and experiences.

3. Take an annual agenda calendar seriously. If you are on a committee, especially if you are a committee chair, ask how the agenda calendar for your committee rolls up into the agenda calendar for the board. Help make the board process productive by being proactive rather than reactive.

4. Regardless of how an item is labeled on an agenda, a CEO or board may treat it as a different type of item. If at any time it is not clear whether the board is receiving information, having a discussion, or making a decision, ask your board chair to clarify.

5. Do not miss the opportunity presented by board retreats. Let your chair and CEO know you consider them a good investment of your time. Help make retreats a valued part of the annual board calendar.

REFERENCES

Bazerman, M. H., and M. D. Watkins. 2004. *Predictable Surprises: The Disasters You Should Have Seen Coming, and How to Prevent Them.* Boston: Harvard Business School Press.

McGinn, P. 2007a. "How to Make a Board Retreat Pay Dividends." *Trustee* 60 (5): 28–29.

———. 2007b. "Making the Case for Conflict." *Trustee* 60 (1): 32, 36.

CHAPTER 12

MAXIMIZING PARTICIPATION AND CONTRIBUTIONS

WHY DO LEADERS and experts in other fields turn into passive bystanders when they serve on healthcare boards? Board members who are astute and articulate in other settings frequently participate less than I expect in board meetings. In "Board Leadership: Who's in the Driver's Seat?" I suggested: "Unfortunately, some healthcare professionals have a tendency to instill doubt and hesitation among board members by implying that healthcare is unique and too complex for a layperson to understand. . . . It is true that many of the rules, regulations, and reimbursement formulas in healthcare are counterintuitive for those accustomed to conventional businesses and professions. Therefore, it is not unusual for board members, who are leaders in other areas, to defer to executives and physicians, who have more familiarity with the jargon, methods, and oddities of healthcare practice and management" (McGinn 2006, 34). CEOs who want active, engaged, and contributing boards must counteract tendencies to instill doubt and hesitation and instead build the knowledge and skills of board members.

BUILDING A KNOWLEDGE BASE

Many board members come to the board with knowledge of general business principles and practices. Some have expertise in organizational development or group process. A few have a background in healthcare. Even fewer have in-depth clinical knowledge. In a board meeting, however, it is likely that issues requiring at least some knowledge in each of these areas will arise. Not every board member needs to be expert in each, but every board member should develop sufficient understanding to follow the discussion, ask reasonable questions, and make prudent decisions.

The best boards develop a learning agenda in response to this uneven knowledge and experience. This typically includes clinical or program presentations at each board meeting, occasional on-site educational sessions, participation in one or more off-site conferences annually, and targeted reading. Some boards subscribe to healthcare-related journals, such as *Trustee* magazine. Unfortunately, the educational agenda is often the first thing to go when the business agenda gets too heavy or board members' personal time gets squeezed by other priorities.

The CEO and board chair need to create a culture of learning. They need to weave learning opportunities into the meeting process and plan education so it follows the *selective* and *just-in-time* principles. The CEO follows the *selective* principle by avoiding the temptation to overwhelm board members with too much of a good thing. Like a good editor, a CEO should select the information that best represents the whole. According to the *just-in-time* principle, presentations, lectures, and readings should be chosen for their relevance to the board's current business agenda. Board members should commit to participating in educational activities and completing the reading. The governance committee can help the CEO plan and implement education to ensure it meets board members' needs.

MENTORING NEW MEMBERS

Many successful people can point to mentors who helped them learn faster, develop skills, make connections, and progress rapidly up their career ladders. We can help others gain these same advantages by assigning mentors who offer advice, connections, and support. Unfortunately, many well-meaning programs have started with this goal and failed because they did not recognize the reciprocal nature of mentoring.

Mentoring relationships arise through positive, two-way interactions. Good mentors understand they have something to offer and feel a responsibility to share it with others. However, they must get something in return: stimulation from teaching an eager learner, fresh insights, or shared energy. There must also be rapport or identification on a personal level.

Although mentoring is a great way to assimilate new board members and prepare them to participate and contribute, assigning each new board member a mentor is not an effective way to make this happen. CEOs will have more success orchestrating rather than assigning mentor relationships. They can start by encouraging senior board members to understand mentoring as one of their roles. Working with their board chairs, CEOs can pair up new board members with senior members for specific tasks, social events, or conferences. They can suggest learning opportunities that specific senior and junior board members might enjoy and benefit from. This allows mentor relationships to develop organically and provides mutually satisfying experiences to mentors and proteges while maximizing board participation and contribution.

Consider the list of dos and don'ts presented in Table 12.1.

DISCUSSION SKILLS

What communication skills do you wish you possessed in greater depth? Public speaking? Persuasiveness? Leading a productive meeting? Inspiring others? Storytelling? What about listening? Listening is the most important yet least developed communication skill. It is what makes a discussion productive. A close cousin to the art of listening is the art of asking good questions—questions

Table 12.1 Creating Effective Mentor Relationships

DO	DON'T
• Coach senior board members to reach out to new board members.	• Name it a mentoring program.
• Pair up complementary individuals on committees or work groups.	• Assume that mentoring comes naturally to everyone or every situation.
• Point out sharing/learning opportunities to individual senior and new board members.	• Assign mentors and mentees, especially on a rotating basis without regard to the individual skills and needs of each mentor and mentee.
• Coach new board members to be responsive and express appreciation when senior board members reach out to them.	• Set it and forget it. Some mentor relationships will root and grow seemingly without effort, but more often nurturing and cultivation are needed.
• Recognize and celebrate new board member contributions and senior member support and guidance.	

that draw out the speaker and help the listener understand more fully what the speaker is saying and why. For example, ask sincerely and without skepticism: "Why do you say that?" "What do you intend by that suggestion?" "How will that work?" In counseling, therapists test their understanding by asking clients confirmatory questions such as: "So, are you saying . . . ?" "Do I understand correctly that you think . . . ?" "It sounds like you are suggesting . . . . Did I get that right?" These approaches translate well to the boardroom. CEOs who model sincere questioning will encourage participation and improve the quality of dialogue.

Another approach that pays off in greater engagement is the "What if?" question. "What if we could only afford to secure one piece of capital equipment above a specific dollar level next year?" "What if we were not so limited by resources?" "What if we were not already providing XYZ service or program?" What-if questions unfreeze thinking. They draw board members into a topic and bring forth new positions and arguments that encourage members to listen to each other.

Table 10.1 identified intrinsic approaches to building trust among board members. One of those was building on ideas, using dialogue such as, "Bill, I like your idea. What would you think if we extended it by combining it with Carl's suggestion?" This reinforces the value of the speaker's message. It also connects board members so discussion benefits from greater continuity and the ideas of several members. The connections are not always obvious, so a listener must attend carefully, find the value in others' comments, and remember them until the opportunity comes to build on them. In a normal group discussion, speakers focus mainly on getting their own ideas across. This leads to discontinuity and a sense of not being heard. When CEOs model building on ideas, their boards arrive at better decisions, feel better about themselves and their colleagues, and adopt the practice themselves.

VALUING DIFFERENCES

"If you and I are always in agreement, one of us is not necessary." I like to refer to this as the first law of diversity (McGinn 2005, 32). In sports and real life, teams and groups perform at higher levels when they have diverse skills and the know-how to capitalize on them. A basketball team composed exclusively of seven-foot centers or speedy, high-scoring point guards would lose to a team that included a balanced array of players.

This principle also applies to boards. This is not immediately apparent because individual roles are not as clearly differentiated in the boardroom as they are on the basketball court. A little reflection, however, reveals the different roles board members play: the historian, the challenger, the conciliator, the devil's advocate, the promoter, the visionary, the conscience, and so on. These roles can be constructive, but they often frustrate board members instead. *Why can't he or she be more like me? Why can't the others see that my ideas are soundest and agree with me?*

CEOs need to recognize differing strengths and model appreciation of them. Many CEOs are familiar with the Myers-Briggs Type Indicator, a personality test commonly used in the workplace. On the Myers-Briggs, there are two perceptual preferences (sensing and intuition) and two judging preferences (thinking and feeling). Although each person has a blend of preferences, one of the four dominates. In Myers-Briggs terms, some board members have greater recognition of and appreciation for facts (sensing), others are more interested in possibilities (intuition), some typically evaluate things logically (thinking), and others make choices from a values orientation (feeling).

These strengths can complement one another in a board setting. Problem solving begins with an understanding of the situation. A senser will ask, "How is this situation similar to others we have faced?" and provide supporting detail. A board member strong on intuition, however, will suggest new ways of approaching the situation, identifying possible targets and alternative proposals. Another board member with a dominant thinking preference will evaluate the options under consideration, using logical criteria like investment, risk, and potential payback. A board member with a feeling preference will evaluate instead how these options fit the mission or values of the organization.

CEOs who carefully watch their boards in action will see different styles and strengths come into play over and over. Board members may pigeonhole each other according to individual differences. In some cases, board members, or even CEOs themselves, may discount in advance the contributions of board members whose style and strengths differ from their own. Like good coaches, however, CEOs need to recognize and value differences and help their boards do the same.

The strongest teams, in sports and in business, possess relevant and diverse talents they can call on as needed. Any board member can spot and encourage diverse talents. Some may be more skilled in this than their CEOs. However, CEOs often have the best vantage point for observing the strengths and input of their board members, so they should take the lead in maximizing board member participation and contribution.

APPLICATION GUIDELINES FOR THE CEO

1. Healthcare is not simple, but avoid making it seem too complex or arcane. You do not want to reduce board members' confidence in their ability to contribute helpfully with their ideas and judgments.
2. Plan board training carefully, using the selective and just-in-time principles to provide the right amount of training when it is needed.
3. Use the list of "dos" in Table 12.1 as a guide to fostering productive mentoring relationships on your board.
4. Model discussion skills, especially listening and building on the ideas of your board members.
5. You are in a unique position to learn the strengths of your board members and deploy them to greatest effect. Do not miss the opportunity to use board members' differences to improve board performance.

APPLICATION GUIDELINES FOR THE BOARD

1. Do not let yourself be intimidated by the jargon or challenges of healthcare management. Creative problem solving often results from coming at old problems from new directions.
2. Commit to learning. Make time to read and participate in voluntary educational opportunities.

3. If you are an experienced board member, reach out to new board members. Let their enthusiasm and freshness rekindle your energy and commitment while you help them become active, contributing members of the board.

4. In board discussions, keep in mind that you can often further discussion more with a good, timely question than with a statement or an assertion.

5. When you find yourself pigeonholing or stereotyping board colleagues, treat it as a signal to raise their strengths to the surface using the discussion skills in this chapter.

REFERENCES

McGinn, P. 2006. "Board Leadership: Who's in the Driver's Seat?" *Trustee* 59 (10): 34.

———. 2005. *Leading Others, Managing Yourself.* Chicago: Health Administration Press.

CHAPTER 13

MAKING DECISIONS

On July 4, 1962, at Independence Hall in Philadelphia, President John F. Kennedy delivered an address on government, independence, and interdependence. Although he spoke about national and global issues, some of his comments apply directly to healthcare organizations and their boards. Kennedy (1962) said, "We are not permitted the luxury of irresolution. Others may confine themselves to debate, discussion, and that ultimate luxury—free advice. Our responsibility is one of decision—for to govern is to choose." CEOs of healthcare organizations will recognize the truth of this statement. Decisions may be difficult, and some executives and boards shy away from them. But making decisions is at the heart of governance. The future of an organization depends on the decisions made today.

ASKING THE RIGHT QUESTIONS

The way a question is *framed* determines the way evidence is gathered, the types of answers that are discovered, and the decisions that result. Consider the story of the CEO who comes upon a man searching for his house keys under a street lamp and offers to help him. After searching fruitlessly for a few minutes, the CEO asks: "Are you sure you dropped them here?" "No," answers the other, pointing to some bushes. "I dropped them over there." "Then why are we looking here?" asks the CEO. "Because this is where the light is," replies the man. It sounds ridiculous, but if you asked some healthcare executives how they measure quality, you might get similar answers. Quality is often defined by the requirements of government reporting, accreditation standards, and public report cards rather than by meaningful data.

Consider the issue of framing from another perspective. In "Manage Your Energy, Not Your Time," Tony Schwartz (2007, 66) says: "It's been a revelation for many of the people we work with to discover they have a choice about how to view a given event. . . . The most effective way people can change a story is to view it through any of three new lenses, which are all alternatives to seeing the world from the victim perspective. With the *reverse lens,* for example, people ask themselves, 'What would the other person in this conflict say and in what ways might that be true?' With the *long lens* they ask, 'How will I most likely view this situation in six months?' With the *wide lens* they ask themselves, 'Regardless of the outcome of this issue, how can I grow and learn from it?'" Different questions can yield different interpretations and different implications.

I also suggest CEOs and boards consider the five types of questions summarized in Table 13.1 to help frame issues and get at the underlying dynamics of any situation. Such questions help CEOs and boards avoid the problem, illustrated by the lost keys story, of accepting the given definition of a challenge without probing more deeply. Good decision making begins with asking good questions. Bad decision making can begin with asking bad questions, but it more often begins with asking no questions at all. Be wary of people who have all the answers, but no questions. They are operating on assumptions, not facts, a stance that is particularly dangerous in a changing environment.

**Table 13.1 Five Types of Questions to Help Frame Issues
for Board Decisions**

	Rationale	Example
Positioning Questions	Identify the current facts (or current position)	"What do the data say about our current levels of patient satisfaction?"
Possibility Questions	Establish targets	"What level of patient satisfaction should we achieve within a year?"
Proposal Questions	Identify options or alternatives	"What approaches do you recommend to move our scores from where they are to where we want them to be?"
Probing Questions	Dig deeper	"Why do you think that approach would yield greater results than our current activities?"
Principle Questions	Tie decision criteria to mission, vision, and values	"Which of these proposals is most consistent with our philosophy of service?"

PLUMBING THE DATA

I had the good fortune to study statistics and experimental design in graduate school with two of the foremost quantitative psychologists of their time, Dr. Warren Torgerson and Dr. Bert Green. Both had national reputations and edited leading journals in the field. What impressed me most, however, was their ability to find the stories that lay within mounds of data. They were never satisfied with standard statistical tests using packaged computerized programs. Instead, they studied data from multiple perspectives until they could discern patterns that revealed new insights.

CEOs and boards should do the same. Rather than accept routine statistics in complex charts and tables, they should try to uncover the real story. For example, in a large medical group, patient satisfaction reports suggested gradual performance improvement across the board. However, when the CFO analyzed the data more carefully, he discovered what was actually happening. One by one, the practice sites were "getting it." When a location "got it," its patient satisfaction score jumped from average or below to outstanding. Therefore, management moved its focus from generic across-the-board training and encouragement to targeted interventions in the lagging practices.

As I explained in Chapter 6, statistics can be used to persuade or mislead. CEOs and board members should be especially skeptical of comparisons to "average" performance. Averages frequently masquerade as facts. Correlations are even more dangerous.

Some numbers are accurate but trivial. Statistical significance tests by themselves have little value for executives. Such tests can determine whether chance is a factor in a controlled experiment, but not whether the results are meaningful in a real-world setting. Be wary of a report with multiple averages and correlations, some of which are significant at the 0.05 or 0.01 level. They won't necessarily teach you anything worthwhile. Do these instead:

- Ask yourself whether the results make sense.
- Ask what story the numbers are telling and what follow-up actions they suggest.
- Ask whether measured differences are large enough to matter.
- Never take a single statistical result as meaningful.
- Remember that a single number never indicates a trend.

Make sure whoever is doing the analysis has looked at the data in at least a couple of different ways. Only when people immerse themselves deeply in the data do they see the connections that lurk beneath the surface. You wouldn't trust a CFO who did not judge the fiscal soundness of an organization on a variety of indexes and ratios. Market share, consumer preferences, patient and employee satisfaction, and quality, among others, are crucial to your mission and long-term success and even less straightforward than finance, so why would you rely on simple indicators? Dig deep. The quality of your decision making depends on it.

IDENTIFYING AND ANALYZING OPTIONS

Anyone who has read *Consumer Reports (CR)* has seen good presentations of decision alternatives and selection criteria. If you are interested in a refrigerator or a flat screen TV, for example, you can consult *CR* and find a chart with different models arrayed across the top and functions or benefits listed in the left column. Each cell of the chart includes a rating indicating each model's performance in each function. This allows a prospective buyer to evaluate multiple options at once and consider trade-offs among the alternatives.

The *Consumer Reports* charts are a variation of a Pugh chart, an evaluation tool used by engineers. Hospital CEOs and board members see similar charts when they evaluate information technology purchases. The Health Care Advisory Board uses them to summarize the results of their benchmarking studies. CEOs would be wise to use such charts for presenting decision choices to their boards.

Without a formal analytical display device, decision-making discussions tend to wander. Substantial research attests to our limited ability to keep more than a handful of facts in active short-term memory or to make multiple discriminations among complex data. When data are displayed in a user-friendly table, however, it is easier for discussion participants to see the forest and the trees—the overview and the specific ratings. CEOs who present decision criteria and data this way will see more productive and focused board discussions.

The use of simple tables and charts in general will pay off in greater board engagement during decision-making discussions. Visual displays of information help CEOs think through issues systematically, locate gaps in information or logic, and complete an analysis board members can understand, build on, and employ in the deliberations. Just as the use of a good metaphor or story encourages listeners to adopt a new framework for understanding a problem, the use of visual decision tools engages board members and helps them consider the choices more logically.

CHOOSING

The structured, systematic approach to analysis and decision making has at least one major problem. An approach that is too mechanical may cost the board the benefits of experience and judgment that are hard to quantify. As Albert Einstein reportedly said, "Not everything that counts can be counted, and not everything that can be counted counts." The board's decision-making responsibility continues to be a profound obligation, even when management has provided complete data and excellent analyses.

How should boards make decisions? Table 13.2 lists alternatives and their advantages and disadvantages. It is not a fully inclusive list. For example, it does not include such traditional favorites as autocratic decisions, sub-group (e.g., executive committee) decisions, and avoidance.

Many people take their preferred methods for granted and do not even consider the alternatives. Groups who typically use majority rule find consensus procedures slow and without rigor. Groups used to unanimity find voting procedures cold

Table 13.2 Alternative Approaches to Decision-Making

Approach	Advantages	Disadvantages
Automatic according to policy (e.g., lowest bidder)	Consistent Fair Quick Simple	Inflexible Sometimes inappropriate Can be gamed May not recognize trade-offs
Logical analysis and voting	Thorough Thoughtful Defensible	May neglect subjective values May miss subtleties May create resistance
Formal approach to approving resolutions (e.g., Robert's rules)	Orderly Clear identification of choice Conflict, if any, can be managed equitably	Subject to parliamentary gamesmanship May be overly formal, or restrictive for the circumstances
Majority voting	Generally perceived as fair Objective Common in American culture	May ignore or disenfranchise minority concerns May achieve premature closure
Supermajority voting (e.g., 2/3 majority)	Generally perceived as fair Objective Less likely to ignore minority concerns	Slower Can frustrate the will of the majority May still override legitimate opposition
Consensus	Assures broad support Allows different styles to affect outcome Avoids premature closure	May be slow May create pressure to conform Outcome may be fuzzy
Unanimity	Signals strong support Forces consideration of all concerns Requires a higher standard of certainty	May be slow A single objector can thwart the will of the many Pressure to conform may be extreme

Table 13.2 *Continued*

Approach	Advantages	Disadvantages
Values-based	May be used in conjunction with any of the above Helps align decisions with organizational or personal mission and values	May reflect biases May be more supportive of the status quo, i.e., "the way we do things." Values can be more difficult to change, even when change is appropriate
Intuition	Calls upon experience or values May encompass broader base of considerations Sensitive to subtle issues	May reflect bias May ignore inconvenient facts or analysis Hard to share/explain to others
Open-ended discussion	Sense of all options being on the table Unlikely but creative options have the opportunity to emerge Lack of pressure	Discussion may replace decision-making Decisions, if any, may be vague and ambiguous Time-consuming

and disenfranchising. Those who use intuition or explicit values to guide decisions clash with those who insist solely on facts and logic.

A CEO helping the board determine what approach fits best in a given circumstance must assess the board's temperament and the stakes involved. Bylaws may call for majority voting or supermajority voting for certain decisions, but that should be only the beginning of the story. There are times when values should be made explicit (e.g., when there is deeply felt conflict over choices). There are times when the merits of intuition may come to the fore (e.g., when considering alternative futures). There are circumstances when calling for a vote will move the board ahead (e.g., when a timely decision is required), but there are other times when slowing down for consensus will unify a board (e.g., when dealing with a sensitive, controversial issue). CEOs and boards should be thoughtful rather than automatic in applying these decision processes.

APPLICATION GUIDELINES FOR THE CEO

1. Decisions are the results of not just facts but also how the facts are framed. Use questions to help your board see issues from multiple perspectives.
2. Be skeptical of staff work that uses many tables and statistics. Look behind the numbers for useful implications. Build organizational capability in statistical analysis.
3. Use visual displays of information. Make them complete enough to be valid, but clear and simple enough that they aid, not confuse, the board.
4. To encourage the board to make decisions, not just engage in discussion, structure the decision-making process with good analytic pre-work and clearly indicate what types of decisions you want.
5. Before each board meeting, confer with your board chair to anticipate what decision-making approach is most appropriate for the issues the meeting will address. Generally, decision making benefits from structure. You must also provide the board with the relevant data and information with sufficient lead time to permit thoughtful review and assessment.

APPLICATION GUIDELINES FOR THE BOARD

1. Recognize when the board is avoiding a decision, and take the initiative to help frame the issue and move toward a decision-making process.

2. Do not always accept the choices presented. Sometimes a good question will reveal different options and better choices.

3. When presented with statistics, always step back and ask if the results make sense. Too many people, CEOs included, accept conclusions as valid just because they are bolstered by numbers. All data need to be interpreted, and there is more than one way to look at any number.

4. Insist alternatives and criteria be presented in a format that aids decision making. Do not accept confusing or partial analyses. If you are confused, do not assume the fault lies in you.

5. Do not accept any single decision-making method as the only valid way. Follow your bylaws, but employ additional approaches to help the board make wise and supportable decisions.

REFERENCES

Kennedy, J. F. 1962. "Address at Independence Hall." [Online article; retrieved 5/30/08.] www.jfklibrary.org/Historical+Resources/Archives/Reference+Desk/Speeches/JFK/003POF03IndependenceHall07041962.htm.

Schwartz, T. 2007. "Manage Your Energy, Not Your Time." *Harvard Business Review* 55 (October): 63–73.

SECTION IV

CHAPTER 14

SYSTEM AND SUBSIDIARY BOARDS

THE FIRST 13 chapters dealt with issues all CEOs face in working toward greater board and organizational effectiveness. This chapter, in contrast, focuses on interactions among related organizations and hence among their respective CEOs and boards. The challenges facing CEOs and boards would be difficult enough if they only had to worry about themselves and their communities. The complexity multiplies, however, for hospitals that are part of systems. Healthcare organizations frequently resemble Russian matryoshka dolls. You look inside one doll or one corporation only to find another. As the number of corporate entities increases, the number of boards and management teams increases, and the number of relationships multiplies.

It is now more common to be part of a system than to be a completely independent, freestanding institution. Economic uncertainties, the need for access to capital, threats from competitors, and the consolidation of payers, among other factors, have made independence unsustainable in many cases while making the potential benefits of scale and economic leverage more compelling. Control and accountability, however, vary greatly among systems, as do the legal structures that bind organizations together. There is no single ideal structure or set of rules for how CEOs and boards should function in such environments. Nevertheless, given the fragmentation of the healthcare delivery industry and the episodic nature of most healthcare delivery, strategic alignment and greater synergy within systems should be a goal.

THE DIFFERENCE BETWEEN THEORY AND PRACTICE

In "Desperately Seeking Synergy," Goold and Campbell (1998) define synergy as the ability of organizations to create more value working together than they could by working apart—through shared knowledge, coordinated strategies, shared resources, vertical integration, combined negotiating power, or the ability to create new business together. More progress has been made toward achieving synergy in the tightly organized health systems I have observed than in loose confederations. However, Goold and Campbell warn that while the benefits of systems may seem obvious, the realities do not always follow the apparent logic.

For example, they suggest system CEOs and boards may suffer from a *parenting bias* and a *skills bias*. Corporate leaders may assume that subsidiary executives who do not jump on the synergy train are being resistant and protecting their home turf. System CEOs are likely to label these subsidiary leaders "parochial" and intervene directly to get them to sign on with the system vision. This is the parenting bias.

Goold and Campbell (1998, 135) also note: "Corporate executives who believe they should intervene are also likely to assume that they have the skills to intervene effectively. All too often, however, they do not. The members of the management team may lack the operating knowledge, personal relationships, or facilitative skills required to achieve meaningful collaboration, or they may simply lack the patience and force of character needed to follow through." This is the skills bias. They acknowledge that systems sometimes need to push members to cooperate—"when, for instance, some units are unaware of promising technical or operational innovations in another unit" (Goold and Campbell 1998, 135)—but contend that intervention should be a last resort.

Just establishing a legal corporate entity and calling it a system does not create synergy. System CEOs and boards need to maintain a sense of balance. Although they have greater legal authority than their subsidiaries, that alone does not imply greater skill, knowledge, or market understanding. On the other hand, in a rapidly changing industry such as healthcare, subsidiary organizations cannot use tradition, past practice, or familiarity to justify resistance to change. Self-interested individuals often undo the promises of synergy to the detriment of the whole. CEOs and boards should focus on another s-word, *symbiosis*, whether between subsidiaries or between a subsidiary and the parent.

COMPETING PERSPECTIVES

Even with good intentions and a spirit of cooperation, the CEOs and boards of systems and subsidiaries often see things differently. Their positions and related responsibilities set up a competition of perspectives. Table 14.1 summarizes these opposing orientations. System executives are responsible for the well-being of the whole, while subsidiary executives and boards are responsible for their own organization first. Accordingly, system executives shift resources to achieve the greatest overall results, for example, moving revenues from mature businesses to invest in growing ones. Subsidiary executives, however, look to maintain control of their own earnings while accessing, if possible, additional financial benefits from the system. The system and its subsidiaries use different stategies: System planning typically stresses strategic fit of the pieces, while subsidiary planning is more likely to emphasize achieving operational successes.

Table 14.1 Typical Differences in Orientation Between System and Subsidiary CEOs

System Orientation	Subsidiary Orientation
Well-being of the system	Well-being of the subsidiary
Strategic fit	Operational effectiveness
Shifting of resources	Control and acquisition of resources
Centralization	Decentralization
Standardization	Flexibility
Control	Freedom
Staff functions	Line functions

As systems grow, they tend toward centralization and standardization. Uniform policies and processes help manage large, complex systems efficiently. Standardization also provides advantages in quality management and performance improvement. Uniformity and control at the system level, however, clash with flexibility and freedom at the subsidiary level. Over time, system-level staff functions seek to organize and control the activities of subsidiary-level line and staff functions. Measurement and reporting systems designed at corporate for implementation in the subsidiaries are signs of this.

System corporations seldom provide direct healthcare services, so staff functions dominate. Line functions dominate within subsidiary organizations because they are in the direct service business and because their staff functions are assumed, at least in part, at the system level. Executives at the two levels often follow different career paths. Miscommunication and mutual misperception can result. Perceived personality conflicts, power grabs, or resistance may just be consequences of different perspectives or a lack of clarity regarding what each entity requires from the other.

I spoke recently with a senior executive of a successful, highly integrated system. He had moved there from another system that was also successful, but much less integrated. He commented that he had always believed trust and a spirit of collaboration were more important than organizational structure. Working in tightly organized and loosely organized systems had led him to revise his opinion. Trust and a spirit of collaboration were essential in either setting, but in the highly integrated system, it was easier to make decisions and move quickly to implement them.

As the CEO of another successful, integrated system said to me, there may be differences of perspective across the system, but there must be alignment on the strategic plan. Every member organization must adopt the system's strategic plan rather than create its own. Multiple perspectives are good, but conflict or unresolved competition make synergy elusive.

MAXIMIZING BENEFITS AND MINIMIZING PROBLEMS

CEOs of systems and subsidiaries need to be clear about their authority. In this instance, what you don't know *can* hurt you. Recently a colleague consulting with several subsidiary CEOs within a system mentioned the system board's ability to hire and fire them. One of the CEOs responded, "No, they can't. Only my own board can do that." His colleagues looked at him in surprise and informed him that the consultant was correct. In that system, the system board, not the subsidiary boards, hired and fired member hospital CEOs. It was in the bylaws, but the CEO had skipped the fine print.

One multi-state system has taken steps to prevent this type of misunderstanding. It has created an authority matrix to spell out who has authority to take what actions. It also notes when system advice and consent are needed and when the system and the local boards hold joint responsibility. Given the turnover of board members and CEOs, this is a useful tool. Even so, mixed authority and responsibility may raise questions. It is not unusual, for example, for the system board to approve budgets while local boards and CEOs are accountable for achieving the budgeted targets.

System and local CEOs should follow three principles:

1. If an authority matrix does not exist, one should be created. System governance is frequently ambiguous. In the creation of a system, intentional ambiguity can prevent objections to consummating the deal. Once the system is in place, however, CEOs will be caught in the crossfire if authority is unclear. If you are a subsidiary CEO, be sure that you, your board chair, and your senior staff understand the extent of your subsidiary's responsibilities and the limits of its authority.

2. Take the initiative in communication. If you are the system CEO, be visible without being domineering. You are the primary spokesperson for the system vision and strategy. It is essential that subsidiary boards understand the system's plans and priorities. If you are a subsidiary CEO, establish a clear, routine dialogue with your system CEO about your board and where it is going. You will need to work together to keep your boards aligned, especially when competitive and financial pressures affect the system and various subsidiaries unevenly.

3. Build an interactive planning process. This calls for candor and assertiveness blended with participation and collaboration. A strictly top-down planning process may look elegant, but it is likely to run into implementation problems. A predominantly bottom-up planning process may stimulate the entrepreneurial energies of subsidiary leaders, but it is likely to waste resources and diminish the system's strategic advantages.

CEOs need to make sure their boards understand their roles within the system. Some CEOs fan the flames of board discontent to justify their own shortcomings or deflect criticism. Working in a system is not easy, and limits on authority almost always chafe CEOs at both levels. Clarity, dialogue, and collaboration are essential.

THE VITAL FEW

CEOs leading complex organizations can adapt models from the computer industry. As Baldwin and Clark (1997) note, innovation in the computer industry accelerated dramatically through the use of modularity. By complying with fundamental principles and design requirements, companies can independently produce complex hardware and software that will function together smoothly.

Baldwin and Clark (1997) identify three elements of modular design:

1. Architecture that specifies what modules will make up a system and what their primary functions will be
2. Interfaces that describe how the parts will interact and communicate
3. Standards that define design rules and how compliance to them will be measured

Within those parameters, module designers are free to innovate. Creating an interlocking system does not require control over all aspects of all pieces, just the vital few: roles, communications, standards, and measurement.

Studies of change and complex adaptive systems have had the same results. Effectiveness does not require precise control over all behavior, only over the key rules or motivators of performance.

A healthcare system that focused on outstanding patient service, for example, discovered that the benefits spread into finance, quality, and employee relations. When the system CEO and subsidiary CEOs saw eye to eye on culture, and when their boards were aligned on principles, power and control issues lessened. The system CEO and parent board set the direction and overall tone, but the subsidiary CEOs and boards enjoyed considerable autonomy in developing plans and taking action that supported and implemented the strategy and culture of the organization.

The risk of miscommunication, ambiguity, and inconsistency is greater when more than one CEO and board are in the mix. Communication, interactive and aligned planning, clear roles, focused measurement, trust, and a collaborative culture are key. These approaches do not eliminate all problems, but they make parenting bias and skills bias less likely. They can offset differences in perspective between system CEOs and subsidiary CEOs. By following the models described in this chapter, CEOs can help their organizations capture at least some of the synergy that system formation promises and help their boards avoid the disappointment caused by frustrated expectations.

APPLICATION GUIDELINES FOR THE CEO

1. As a CEO within a system, you will be under pressure to achieve synergy. This is reasonable and expected. Do not let yourself or your board fall victim to the mentality that the system is always right—or always wrong.

2. Anticipate normal differences in perspective between the system and subsidiaries. These will be most severe when resources are tight. Differences are often misdiagnosed as personality conflicts, power grabs, or resistance. These things may happen, but do not automatically assume they are the most likely explanations for problems you observe.

3. Know your bylaws. Know where authority and responsibility lie. It will not always be where you expect.

4. Make sure your board knows where system board and subsidiary board authority and responsibility lie. In systems, these areas can get murky.

5. Plan to spend even more time than you would ordinarily expect on role definition, interactive planning, and development of shared values. Make sure each entity can identify benefits of its association with the other. This will lessen frustrations while increasing opportunities for synergy.

APPLICATION GUIDELINES FOR THE BOARD

1. Do not expect synergy to come easily even if logic supports the value of system integration. Work with your CEO to achieve a suitable integration level.

2. Keep your fiduciary responsibilities in mind and insist on open dialogue to ensure that you create and support win-win strategies for the system and its subsidiaries.

3. Ask for an authority matrix. If there is ambiguity, clear it up. Some ambiguity is acceptable if there are sufficient resources, good will, common culture, and shared objectives to balance it. If any of these is missing, lack of clarity may lead to conflict and frustration.

4. Be wary when executives blame their system or subsidiary counterparts for performance shortcomings. They might be right, but do not blindly accept it.

5. Insist CEOs share the architecture of the system, a description of key interfaces, and the standards or principles for communication and interaction. Otherwise, these may remain implicit or assumed.

REFERENCES

Baldwin, C. Y., and K. B. Clark. 1997. "Managing in an Age of Modularity." *Harvard Business Review* 75 (September–October): 84–93.

Goold, M., and A. Campbell. 1998. "Desperately Seeking Synergy." *Harvard Business Review* 76 (September–October): 131–43.

CHAPTER 15

CONCLUSION

As I BEGAN this book, I happened on a sight that made me stop and think once again about why some organizations succeed while others fail. My daughter and I were driving to a store in South Philadelphia adjacent to the Delaware River. As she parked the car, I glanced across the street. There was a huge, rusting ocean liner tied to a dock—the SS *United States*, the "Big U."

I had not seen the Big U in person since I sailed on it as a crewmember in the summer of 1967. From bow to stern, the ship stretches longer than three football fields, and it weighs more than 50,000 tons. On its maiden voyage, it set the speed record for a transatlantic crossing by a commercial vessel. The SS *United States* had once been a great ocean liner.

Working on the Big U was quite an education, but some of the most valuable lessons were in how *not* to manage. The SS *United States* was grossly overstaffed. There was a huge gulf between officers and crew. We were not aligned. We were proud to sail on such an impressive vessel and boasted about it when we were in port, but we were living off past glories, not adding to them.

The fastest ocean liner afloat stopped sailing for good in 1969. It has been tied up in South Philly for years, rusting while it waits for a second chance. Although I had not seen the SS *United States* in 40 years, I had often thought about it as I considered management and leadership issues. Any organization that measures the wrong things; has a disengaged work force and an aloof, invisible leadership; and rests on its reputation and past accomplishments could suffer the same fate. The Big U is as sad to look at now as it was impressive then.

Many hospitals bear a surface resemblance to the Big U. They have large, impressive facilities. Their communities point to them with pride. They employ many people. Their futures seem assured. But 40 years from now, could we drive into communities where hospitals are flourishing today and find boarded-up buildings that no longer serve a purpose because management, staff, and board became complacent or disconnected? The cruise ship industry is flourishing, but the SS *United States* is not. Could that happen to your organization? Success and survival are not guaranteed even for organizations providing essential community services.

CEO AS CONSULTANT

In the introduction, I suggested that CEOs emulate consultants to constructively engage their boards and make them more effective. Throughout the book, I have pointed out ways CEOs can coach and advise board members while respecting their different roles and responsibilities.

For example, in helping their boards select new members, CEOs should look at their boards' current and future challenges and advise them regarding the criteria and candidates that would best serve their needs. This means CEOs must take the long view and carefully analyze alternatives. Likewise, CEOs can coach physicians and other board members who are impatient and irritated with board processes. Just as consultants would, CEOs can provide private insights and suggest ways board members can work together more effectively. They can guide board members through the complexities of healthcare to their joint advantage and to the benefit of the organization as a whole.

Occasionally, CEOs may find themselves in conflict with their boards or may observe disagreements among board members. CEOs, acting as consultants to their boards, can raise issues respectfully for mutual consideration and candid dialogue. They can bring hidden agendas and unspoken objectives into the open. CEOs benefit from clarifying expectations. Moreover, CEOs following the consultant model will engage in two-way communication with their boards to ensure trust and mutual understanding and to build the board's knowledge base and confidence. Without these, boards may make either of two common errors: intervening when inappropriate or not demonstrating leadership when their active involvement is needed.

The size and complexity of healthcare organizations place enormous stress on trustees. Hospital trustees are not born understanding how these institutions work, nor in most cases have they received specialized training. Nevertheless, they are responsible for the fiscal soundness of the organizations and the quality of care provided. CEOs should recognize their responsibility to make sure their boards are up to the challenge.

STRATEGY

Chapter 5, the first chapter about what boards do, focuses on defining purpose and setting direction. Without a shared understanding of mission and vision, organizations cannot capitalize on their human and financial resources. CEOs who wish to engage their boards productively should begin with mission, vision, values, and strategy.

Survival is not guaranteed for not-for-profit healthcare organizations. They face financial, competitive, and regulatory pressures. It is easy for CEOs and boards to get distracted and to lose perspective. CEOs serve their boards, their communities, and their organizations well by continuing to move forward in the face of obstacles and challenges.

Boards sometimes take a passive role in strategic planning, however. As Chait, Ryan, and Taylor (2005) point out, boards may treat strategic planning like they do budgets: CEOs propose strategies, which boards review, discuss, and vote on, usually with minimal changes. They suggest CEOs create strategy *with* their boards rather than *for* their boards. CEOs and boards should articulate a shared vision to sharpen the focus for organizational investment and actions. Boards should neither defer to management nor dominate in the definition of the mission, vision, values, and strategy of the organization. These should be collaborative activities.

RELATIONSHIPS

Chapter 10, the first chapter about how boards should do their work, focuses on relationships. My early work with total quality management taught me that the quality of relationships within a team predicted the team's success. I learned that teams who were completely task focused and got down to work immediately were *less* successful than teams who attended to relationships and spent time getting to know each other as individuals and building a sense of themselves together as a team.

The time to build trust and respect is *before* they are needed. CEOs should develop strong relationships while things are progressing well. When the inevitable problems arise, board members will already have the necessary mutual regard to work together effectively. Board members must be willing to stand by their organizations and each other rather than scatter when the first strong pressures hit them. CEOs who build or enhance personal relationships among board members will be rewarded by their boards' strength in times of crisis. When board members develop mutual trust and respect, it is like weaving the cables of a bridge. Their combined strength is far greater than the strength of the individual components. As Sonnenfeld (2002) concludes, what makes great boards great is not rules and regulations; it is the way people work together.

THE ROAD AHEAD

My dog, Riley, is a bit smarter than the average dog, but he's also a lot more stubborn—certainly more stubborn than smart. When I take him on long walks, he often reaches a point where he wants to go no further. He drags behind me, he pants, he lets his tongue hang out and his tail droop, and he gives a convincing impression that he is physically spent. Sometimes he will do this on a circular walk when we are well past the halfway point. Nothing will get him to move ahead. To an outside observer, it looks like I have pushed this poor dog to exhaustion. If I relent and turn around, however, his tail curls back up, the spring returns to his step, and he happily retraces his steps back to our starting point.

A CEO happened to call my cell phone during a recent walk, just as Riley had decided to go no further. As we talked, I described Riley's behavior. He replied, "There's a management story there." He was right: One of the challenges of leadership is the need to move forward, even when the road ahead is uncertain and the road behind is comfortable and familiar.

I wrote about the dangers of complacency for healthcare executives in an earlier book (McGinn 2005), in a chapter titled "If You Are Coasting, You Are Going Downhill." CEOs and boards sometimes seek the comfort of the familiar instead of driving forward to achieve their organizational missions. CEOs need to recognize when they, their boards, or their organizations are coasting. They need to remember their roles as keepers and promoters of the vision. When people want to turn back, CEOs must inspire the board and staff to overcome obstacles and stay focused on mission and strategy.

This chapter should not be considered the end. No value comes from reading this book unless it leads to taking action. The demands on CEOs are great, but CEOs are not alone. Their boards can be their partners and collaborators and can help them achieve more for their organizations and communities than they possibly could on their own.

APPLICATION GUIDELINES FOR THE CEO

1. (Chapter 1) As CEO, and as a partner of the board, you should have great interest in getting the right people on the bus as board members. You should encourage and facilitate board self-evaluation and ensure that proper attention and lead time are provided for the nomination process. You can recommend processes, identify role models, suggest educational opportunities, and propose schedules that help the board fulfill this responsibility. That is part of your "consulting" role. The quality of your relationship with your board chair will be a major factor in your ability to advance these ideas.

2. (Chapter 3) The responsibilities of board chair weigh heavily on many who take the role. You do both of yourselves a favor when you mentor your "boss." Providing support and affirmation reduces stress, especially early on. Never doubt that the selection of the board chair is critical. Do not settle for compromises. Be aware that if you and the chair do not groom upcoming leaders, the board's choices for future leadership may be limited.

3. (Chapter 5) Passion drives excellence. Boards can lose their sense of passion and mission because they are so far from the organization's actual service delivery. When you help the board stay focused on purpose, you help sustain their passion and commitment. When you focus only on survival, the organization settles for mediocrity rather than striving for excellence.

4. (Chapter 9) Humans and their organizations seek comfortable equilibrium, so problems are often fixed only temporarily, until people revert back to their old habits. If you do not build tracking mechanisms to ensure lasting change, you will find yourself dealing with the same problems again and again and losing credibility with your board.

5. (Chapter 12) You are in a unique position to learn the strengths of your board members and deploy them to greatest effect. Do not miss the opportunity to use board members' differences to improve board performance.

APPLICATION GUIDELINES FOR THE BOARD

1. (Chapter 1) Focus first on the mission of the organization and then on the results that are achieved by management and the medical staff. As not-for-profit board members, you are the trustees of the community's interests. Focusing on the mission will ensure that you do not get sidetracked into administrative work or responsibilities. Your passion for the mission will be a great attractor for the people you want on board. Focusing on outcomes will fulfill the responsibilities to the community you have as board members.

2. (Chapter 3) Board leadership brings many responsibilities. Do not select people for leadership and then abandon them. Volunteer to help; do not delegate up.

3. (Chapter 4) Increase the vitality of board meetings by interacting directly with other board members in discussion: Ask questions, build on comments, support good ideas, raise alternatives, and challenge perceptions. This helps the CEO maintain an appropriate activity level in board meetings.

4. (Chapter 9) Make sure you speak up early about the results most important to you as a board. This will help with selecting the right measures, and you will know when organizational efforts hit or miss.

5. (Chapter 5) Many boards defer to management in the articulation of the mission, vision, values, and strategy of the organization. Do not defer. Do not dominate. Be a partner. Collaborate.

REFERENCES

Chait, R. P., W. P. Ryan, and B. E. Taylor. 2005. *Governance as Leadership: Reframing the Work of Nonprofit Boards*. Hoboken, NJ: John Wiley & Sons.

McGinn, P. 2005. *Leading Others, Managing Yourself*. Chicago: Health Administration Press.

Sonnenfeld, J. 2002. "What Makes Great Boards Great." *Harvard Business Review* 80 (September): 106–13.

Index

ABOUT THE AUTHOR

Peter McGinn, PhD, is the founder and president of Leadership Impact, LLC, a consulting practice that helps leaders and organizations excel by bringing out the best in people and aligning their talents with the goals of their organizations. He is also a senior advisor for Health Strategies and Solutions, a leading national healthcare consulting firm. Prior to founding Leadership Impact in 2007, Dr. McGinn served for seven years as CEO of United Health Services in Binghamton, New York. Previously, Dr. McGinn has worked as a vice president of the Johns Hopkins Health System and as a hospital psychologist.

Dr. McGinn is the author of *Leading Others, Managing Yourself*, published by Health Administration Press, and *Learning to Lead*, an American College of Healthcare Executives self-study course. He has also written articles on board leadership for *Trustee* magazine and on executive skills for *Hospitals and Health Networks OnLine*. He is a frequent speaker and facilitator for executive and board training and work sessions.

Dr. McGinn received his PhD in psychology from Johns Hopkins. He is past chair of HANYS, the Healthcare Association of New York State. He received the Distinguished Service Award from HANYS in 2007.